Management of
PSORIASIS

Management of
PSORIASIS

Neena Khanna MD
Professor and Head
Department of Dermatology
Amrita Institute of Medical Sciences and Research Centre
Faridabad, Haryana, India

Sachin Gupta MD
Senior Resident
Department of Dermatology
Amrita Institute of Medical Sciences and Research Centre
Faridabad, Haryana, India

Bela Bhat MD
Assistant Professor
Department of Dermatology
Amrita Institute of Medical Sciences and Research Centre
Faridabad, Haryana, India

Vichitra MD
Senior Resident
Department of Dermatology
Amrita Institute of Medical Sciences and Research Centre
Faridabad, Haryana, India

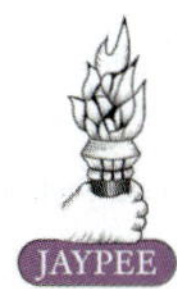

JAYPEE BROTHERS MEDICAL PUBLISHERS
The Health Sciences Publisher
New Delhi | London

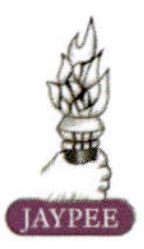 **Jaypee Brothers Medical Publishers (P) Ltd**

Headquarters

EMCA House
23/23-B, Ansari Road, Daryaganj
New Delhi 110 002, India
Landline: +91-11-23272143, +91-11-23272703
+91-11-23282021, +91-11-23245672
E-mail: jaypee@jaypeebrothers.com

Corporate Office

Jaypee Brothers Medical Publishers (P) Ltd.
4838/24, Ansari Road, Daryaganj
New Delhi 110 002, India
Phone: +91-11-43574357
Fax: +91-11-43574314
E-mail: jaypee@jaypeebrothers.com

Overseas Office

JP Medical Ltd.
83, Victoria Street, London
SW1H 0HW (UK)
Phone: +44-20 3170 8910
Fax: +44(0)20 3008 6180
E-mail: info@jpmedpub.com

Website: www.jaypeebrothers.com
Website: www.jaypeedigital.com

Management of Psoriasis / *Neena Khanna, Sachin Gupta, Bela Bhat, Vichitra*

First Edition: **2025**

ISBN: 978-93-5696-767-0

Printed in India at Sterling Graphics Pvt. Ltd.

Preface

Psoriasis significantly impacts quality of life, demanding effective and diverse treatment strategies. This edition of *"Management of Psoriasis,"* authored by Dr Neena Khanna, Dr Bela Bhat, Dr Sachin Gupta, and Dr Vichitra from the Department of Dermatology at Amrita Institute of Medical Sciences and Research Centre, Faridabad, Haryana, India, delivers concise, practical guidance on managing psoriasis. Our approach, inspired by the compassionate teachings of Mata Amritanandamayi (Amma), emphasizes holistic and empathetic patient care, integrating a broad spectrum of treatment options.

This book is designed as a to-the-point resource, offering dermatologists, researchers, and students quick access to comprehensive treatment protocols. By providing a thorough overview of available treatments in a practical format, we aim to enhance patient outcomes and support dermatology professionals in their clinical practice.

Neena Khanna
Sachin Gupta
Bela Bhat
Vichitra

Acknowledgments

We owe a debt of gratitude to our entire team of the Department of Dermatology at Amrita Institute of Medical Sciences and Research Centre, Faridabad, Haryana, India, for their invaluable contributions to this edition of *"Management of Psoriasis"*. We are thankful for the support and expertise provided by our fellow coauthors and colleagues, which have been instrumental in crafting a comprehensive guide to psoriasis management.

We are especially grateful to our families and loved ones for their understanding, patience, and encouragement during the writing of this book. Without their unwavering support, this project would not have been possible.

We would like to extend special thanks to our clinical and administrative staff, especially our patient care coordinators and nursing staff, whose diligent work behind the scenes ensures the smooth operation of our department and facilitates our research and clinical endeavors. Their unwavering support and commitment are fundamental to our success and deeply appreciated.

We are deeply grateful to the publishing team at Jaypee Brothers Medical Publishers (P) Ltd, New Delhi, India, especially Nedup Bhutia Pillai (Assistant Manager—Print Publishing) and Ankit Singh (Commissioning Editor). Despite our team missing multiple deadlines and often requesting additional time, their patience and professionalism never wavered. Their understanding and support were instrumental in bringing this edition to fruition. Thank you for accommodating our needs with such grace and dedication.

Finally, we acknowledge the patients themselves, whose experiences and challenges with psoriasis inspire our continuous pursuit of knowledge and more effective treatments. This book is ultimately for you, and it is your journey that motivates us to improve and refine our approach to care.

Neena Khanna
Sachin Gupta
Bela Bhat
Vichitra

Contents

Section 1

Pathogenesis and Clinical Features

Epidemiology

Introduction

Psoriasis is a chronic skin disease characterized by the presence of papules and plaques that are:

- Well-defined
- Erythematous
- Scaly

Relapses and remissions are common in psoriasis: 40–55% of patients report spontaneous remissions for variable lengths of time. Management of the disease requires knowledge not only of the therapeutic modalities available but also its epidemiology, causative, and aggravating factors and behavior in different individuals as well as its impact on patients' quality of life.

Epidemiology of Psoriasis

Prevalence

- Global prevalence of psoriasis varies from 0.09% to 11.4%, indicating that it is a common dermatosis.
- Prevalence is higher in colder climates of UK (1.6%), Norway (1.4%), and USA (4.6%) and is maximum in Arctic region of USSR (11%).
- In India, prevalence of psoriasis varies from 0.44 to 2.8%.

Sex

Psoriasis affects both sexes, almost equally.

Age

Psoriasis can begin at any age. Age of onset of chronic plaque psoriasis has a bimodal distribution:

- *Early onset or type I*, which is characterized by:
  - Onset in second decade
  - Positive family history
  - Frequent association with Human Leukocyte Antigen (HLA)-Cw6
  - Severe disease, with more arthropathy
  - Prominent Koebner's phenomenon
  - Prolonged course, requiring relatively more aggressive therapy.
- *Late onset or type II*, which is characterized by:
  - Onset in fifth decade
  - Relatively milder course
  - Guttate psoriasis is a disease of adolescence.

Race

Racial variation has been described:
- Low incidence in West Africans and Japanese
- Very low incidence in North and South American-Indians.

Pathogenesis

Introduction

Psoriasis is a *T-cell-centered disorder*. Cytokines released from activated T cells as well as other cells:

- Increase the proliferation of keratinocytes.
- Are chemotactic for neutrophils and lymphocytes.
- Are responsible for angiogenesis.

Patients inherit the predisposition to develop psoriasis, but the disease manifests only after being triggered by certain exogenous/antigenic factors.

Genetic Factors

The genetic hypothesis is supported by:

- A strong familial association of the disease. If both parents have psoriasis, offspring have a 50% chance of developing it. With one affected parent, the child's risk drops to 16%. If a child has psoriasis with unaffected parents, siblings face an 8% risk.
- Twin studies have shown a 35–73% concordance for psoriasis among pairs of monozygotic twins but only 12–22% concordance among dizygotic twins.
- Strong association with human leukocyte antigen (HLA) class I and II antigens: HLA-B13, B17, B39, B57, Cw6, Cw7, DR4, and DR7.
- Of these, *HLA-Cw6* shows the highest risk for the early development of psoriasis and *HLA-B27* has risk for psoriatic arthropathy.

Gene Loci

The inheritance of predisposition to develop psoriasis is polygenic.

- At least nine different psoriasis susceptibility loci (PSORS 1-9) have been identified in genome linkage scans. These loci are situated on different chromosomes[1] and are the major genetic determinants for psoriasis, accounting for 30–50% of the heritability of the disease. The two important loci include:
  - A locus for psoriasis susceptibility, within the major histocompatibility complex (MHC) region of chromosome 6p21. This is the locus where several other genes[2] involved in immune regulation are also located.
  - A locus for psoriatic arthritis susceptibility, on the distal end of the long arm of human chromosome 17q25.
- Three genes standout as potential psoriasis susceptibility genes: *HLA-C, HCR,* and *corneodesmosin.*

Environmental Factors

Though patients inherit the predisposition to develop psoriasis, the disease manifests only after being triggered by certain environmental/antigenic factors. A number of triggering factors have been identified discussed further.

Trauma

- Lesions can develop at sites of physical injuries like burns, cuts (including surgical incisions), and scratches.
- This phenomenon is called *Koebner's phenomenon* or *isomorphic phenomenon.*[3]
- It indicates disease activity.

---

[1] *Chromosomes:* 6p21, 17q24-q25, 1q21.3, 3q21, 16q12-q13, and 4q28-q31 have been identified.

[2] These include the gene encoding CD7 (a T lymphocyte Ag expressed on peripheral T cells), the gene encoding intercellular adhesion molecule-2 (ICAM-2), I-309 gene (which encodes a protein produced by activated T lymphocytes) and interleukin (IL) enhancer binding factor gene.

[3] *Isomorphic:* Similar morphology, in contrast to isotopic; meaning similar site.

Climate

- Cold climate and low humidity are associated with aggravation of the disease.
- Hot sunny climate and high humidity are associated with improvement of psoriasis.

Infections

- Bacterial infections, especially streptococcal infections of upper respiratory tract, are known to precipitate guttate psoriasis.
- Infections can also precipitate other types of psoriasis.[4] Bacterial endotoxins are thought to act as superantigens and through the process of antigenic mimicry, activate T-lymphocytes, macrophages, and Langerhans' cells.
- Infection with human immunodeficiency virus may be associated with onset of explosive psoriasis.

Drugs

Several drugs can precipitate psoriasis and pustular psoriasis **(Table 2.1)**. Similarly, withdrawal of systemic corticosteroids can precipitate psoriasis, including pustular psoriasis.

Addictions

- *Alcohol*: It is thought to exacerbate psoriasis and an increased intake of alcohol is often associated with severe forms of the disease.
- *Smoking*: It is alleged to increase the risk of developing psoriasis and pustular psoriasis of palms/soles.

Stress

- Emotional stress is known to aggravate psoriasis. It is more evident in some patients and is probably related to the patient's innate inability to cope with stress.
- Psoriasis itself is a stress-inducing disease and affects the patient's quality of life.

---

[4] This is the rationale for some dermatologists regularly using antimicrobials to treat chronic plaque psoriasis.

TABLE 2.1: Drugs[5] which precipitate/aggravate psoriasis.	
Psoriasis	• ACE inhibitors • Antimalarials • Beta-blockers • Lithium • Nonsteroidal anti-inflammatory agents • Immune checkpoint inhibitors • TNF inhibitors[1]
Pustular psoriasis	• Amiodarone • Atenolol • Calcipotriol • Hydroxychloroquine • Interferon alpha • Lithium • Morphine • Penicillin • Phenylbutazone • Potassium iodide • Procaine • Propranolol • Salicylates • Sulfonamides

(ACE: angiotensin-converting enzyme; TNF: tumor necrosis factor)

Immune Mechanism in Psoriasis

Several observations point toward an immune mechanism in pathogenesis of psoriasis:

- Linkage between HLA antigens[6] and psoriasis
- Spontaneous remissions and exacerbation of the disease activity support an ongoing immune mechanism. Chronicity of the disease suggests existence of memory cells.
- Effectiveness of immunosuppressive drugs like cyclosporine A, methotrexate, corticosteroids, and photochemotherapy.

---

[5] Paradoxically, TNF inhibitors, used for treatment of psoriasis, can occasionally result in psoriasis-like lesions.

[6] There is a strong association between psoriasis and HLA class I and II Ags: HLA-B13, B17, B39, B57, B6, Cw6, Cw7, DR4, and DR7. Of these, HLA-Cw6 shows the highest risk for the development of psoriasis.

Dysregulation of the skin immune system[7] is implicated in the development of psoriasis. This involves an intricate interaction between the keratinocytes, dendritic cells, T cells, keratinocytes, and neutrophils. Cytokines released by these cells are responsible for initiation and maintenance of cutaneous inflammation responsible for psoriasis.

Role of Innate Immunity

Role of T Cells

Psoriasis is a T-cell-mediated disease driven to some extent by a positive feedback loop from activated T cells to antigen-presenting cells (APCs) that is mediated by interferon gamma (IFN-γ), IL-1, and tumor necrosis factor-α (TNF-α). Moreover, there are important contributions of innate immune mechanisms involving the epidermis and macrophages. In psoriatic legions, there is a distinct compartmentalization of T-cells between the anatomic layers of the skin: CD4+ T cells are found predominantly in the upper dermis, whereas CD8+ T cells mostly localize to the epidermis. The functional importance of T-cells is emphasized by the high therapeutic efficacy of cyclosporine A, a T-cell-selective immunosuppressant, as well as other T-cell selective immunomodulators, including anti-CD4 antibodies, CTLA4lg, alefacept, and DAB389IL-2. Biologics that block TNF-α are also highly effective, reflecting important roles for this multifunctional cytokine in antigen (Ag) presentation, macrophage activation, and leukocyte trafficking.

The T-cells in psoriasis can be activated both:

- In the absence of Ag, most importantly by cytokines released by injured keratinocytes.
- In the presence of Ag, either by conventional Ags or bacterial superantigens.

Activation of T-lymphocytes in Absence of Antigens

In genetically predisposed individuals, keratinocytes, on being injured, secrete several cytokines, which activate T-lymphocytes

---

[7] *Skin immune system*: It consists of lymphocytes, antigen-presenting cells (including both HLA DR+ CD1+ Langerhans cells and HLA DR+ CD1–non-Langerhans cells), and keratinocytes.

which in turn initiate and sustain the psoriatic process. The cytokines secreted by keratinocytes include:

- *IL-1*: It has the following actions:
  - ○ Induces keratinocyte proliferation.
  - ○ Stimulates the production of chemotactic cytokines, like IL-8.
  - ○ Induces adhesion molecules.
- *IL-6, IL-7, and IL-8*: These are potent T-cell and neutrophil chemotactic factors, responsible for the formation of Munro's microabscesses.
- *IL-10*: Downregulated
- *TNFα*: It is a central cytokine in pathogenesis of psoriasis and has the following actions:
  - ○ Induces IL-8 (potent chemotactic agent).
  - ○ Upregulates ICAM-1 expression in vascular cells to facilitate lymphocyte trafficking.
  - ○ Induces transforming growth factor beta (TGF-β).
- *Growth factors*: These include TGF-α and β, which stimulate proliferation of keratinocytes, and promote production of vascular endothelial growth factor/vascular permeability factor (VEGF/VPF) to promote angiogenesis and vascular hyperpermeability.

Activation of T-lymphocytes in Presence of Antigens

T-lymphocytes can be persistently stimulated and activated by a variety of Ags:

- *Unidentified conventional Ags*: These antigens are presented to T-lymphocytes by APCs in epidermis and dermis.
- *Bacterial superantigens*: These antigens initiate the process of antigenic mimicry between bacterial proteins (e.g., *Streptococcus*) and type-1 keratin proteins (keratin 17), thereby activating specific T-cells, resulting in autoimmunity.

The Ag-activated T-cells in turn release:

- Various cytokines[8] such IL-2, IL-6, and IL-8 which directly stimulate keratinocyte proliferation.
- INF-α that upregulates ICAM-1 expression by both keratinocyte and endothelial cells.

Recently new subsets of human T-cells expressing IL-17 and IL-22 have been postulated to play a key role in the pathogenesis

---

[8] Because of predominant expression of IL-2 and INF and the lack of IL-4 in the skin lesions, psoriasis is believed to be characterized by a Th1 response.

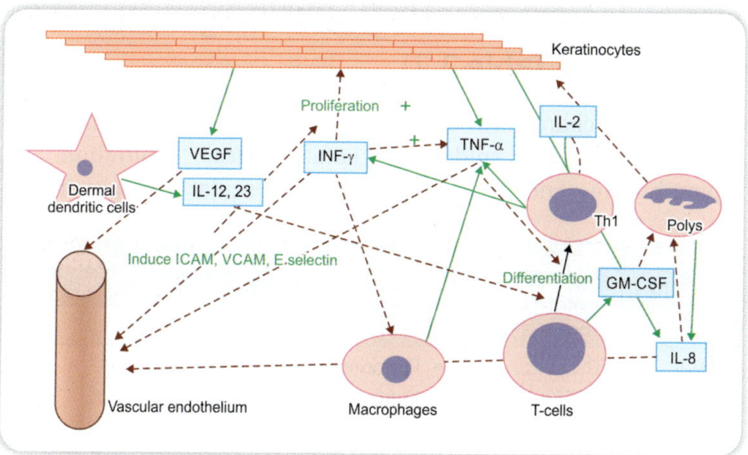

Fig. 2.1: Immunologic pathogenesis of psoriasis: The key cells include Th1 cells, dermal dendritic cells, polymorphs, and macrophages.

(GM-CSF: granulocyte-macrophage colony-stimulating factor; INF: interferon; ICAM: intercellular adhesion molecule; IL: interleukin; TNF: tumor necrosis factor; VCAM: vascular cell adhesion molecule; VEGF: vascular endothelial growth factor)

of psoriasis. Expansion and survival of these cells is driven by IL-23 produced by dendritic APCs acting on IL-23 receptors on T-cells. IFN-γ causes APCs to produce IL-1 and IL-23 and stimulating expansion of IL-17+ and IL-22+ CD8+ T-cells in psoriasis lesions **(Fig. 2.1)**. There is no overlap between T-cells expressing IL-17 and those expressing IL-22 in normal or psoriatic skin and these cells form an important link in the chain connecting genetics and immunology of psoriasis.

Keratinocytes in turn are stimulated to secrete their own cytokines to maintain the psoriatic process.

Role of Keratinocytes

There is an intimate interaction between T-lymphocytes and keratinocytes.

- In predisposed individuals, keratinocytes release cytokines (IL-6, 7, and 8) in response to trauma. These cytokines stimulate T-cells and are chemotactic for polymorphs.
- And in turn, cytokines (IL-2, IL-6, and IL-8) released by lymphocytes stimulate keratinocyte proliferation.

Summary of Immunological Pathogenesis (Fig. 2.1 and Table 2.2)

Psoriasis is characterized by hyperproliferation and abnormal differentiation of epidermal keratinocytes, infiltration by T-lymphocytes and various endothelial vascular changes in the

TABLE 2.2: Immunologic pathogenesis of psoriasis: The key cytokines include TNF-α, IFN-γ, and IL.

Cytokines	Source(s)	Effects
TNF-α	Th1 cells, macrophages, keratinocytes	• Promotes Th1 differentiation • Induces ICAM, VCAM, and E selection
IFN-γ	Th1 cells	Keratinocyte proliferation; increases MHC I and II expression; Ag presentation, attracts macrophages and release of TNF-α; induces ICAM, VCAM, and E selection; inhibits IL-4 (and Th2 expression)
IL-2	Th1 cells	Promotes CD28-CD80-CD86 interaction and clonal proliferation of Th1 cells; activates macrophages and Th1
IL-3	T-cells	Growth of dendritic cells and macrophages
IL-12	APC	Promotes Th1 differentiation
IL-8	Neutrophils, keratinocytes	Attracts lymphocytes and neutrophils; induces vascular response
IL-17	Th17 cells	Drives keratinocyte proliferation and immune cells production of neutrophil-attracting chemokines
IL-23	Antigen presenting cells	Induction, expansion, maintenance, and downstream effector functions of Th17 and Th22 cells
GM CFS	T-cells	Activates neutrophils and mononuclear cells
VEGF	Keratinocytes	Promotes angiogenesis
RANTES	Keratinocytes	Induces IL-12; attracts lymphocytes
MIG, IP-10	Keratinocytes	Increases leukocyte adhesion

(Ag: antigen; APC: antigen presenting cells; GM CSF: granulocyte-macrophage colony-stimulating factor; ICAM: intercellular adhesion molecule; IFN: interferon; IL: interleukin; IP-10: interferon gamma-induced protein 10; MHC: major histocompatibility complex; MIG: monokine induced by gamma interferon; RANTES: regulated on activation, normal T cell expressed and secreted; Th1 cells: type 1 helper T cells; TNF: tumor necrosis factor; VCAM: vascular cell adhesion molecule; VEGF: vascular endothelial growth factor)

dermis. These changes can be explained on the basis of three basic events mediated by cytokines:

1. *Epidermal proliferation*: There is rapid proliferation and maturation of epidermal cells due to an increase in the proliferating cell compartment (basal/suprabasal epidermis) mediated by TGF-β, IFN-γ, and other cytokines (IL-1, IL-2, IL-6, and IL-8). This manifests as:
   i. Shortened epidermal cell cycle with the basal cells going through the process of keratinization and *cornification* in 1.5 days (normal, 13 days).
   ii. Faster maturation and shedding of epidermal cells in 4 days (normal, 26 days).
2. *Marked dermal angiogenesis*: Due to mediators released primarily by keratinocytes, e.g., VEGF and TGF-α.
3. *Munro's microabscesses*: Mediated by chemotactic effect of IL-8.

Mucocutaneous Manifestations

Introduction

The clinical presentation of psoriasis is better understood when it is realized that disease activity can range from a chronic stationary phase to acute episodes of flares, to periods of remissions.

Onset

Two patterns of onset of psoriasis are recognized:
1. *Chronic*:
    i. Seen in about 85% of patients with psoriasis.
    ii. Morphological prototype is chronic plaque psoriasis.
    iii. Lesions appear slowly, increase in size and number, over time.
    iv. Course is punctuated with episodes of relapses and periods of remissions as well as acute episodes.
2. *Acute*: Two morphological patterns show an acute onset:
    i. Guttate psoriasis
    ii. Pustular psoriasis

Morphology

Common Features

The lesions of psoriasis are characteristic and show the following features:
- Are sharply demarcated (**Fig. 3.1**), mildly indurated plaques.
- Are surmounted with nonadherent, lamellar silvery scales (**Fig. 3.2**). If scales are minimal, they can be accentuated by scraping the lesions with a glass slide *(Grattage test)*.
- Positive Auspitz sign

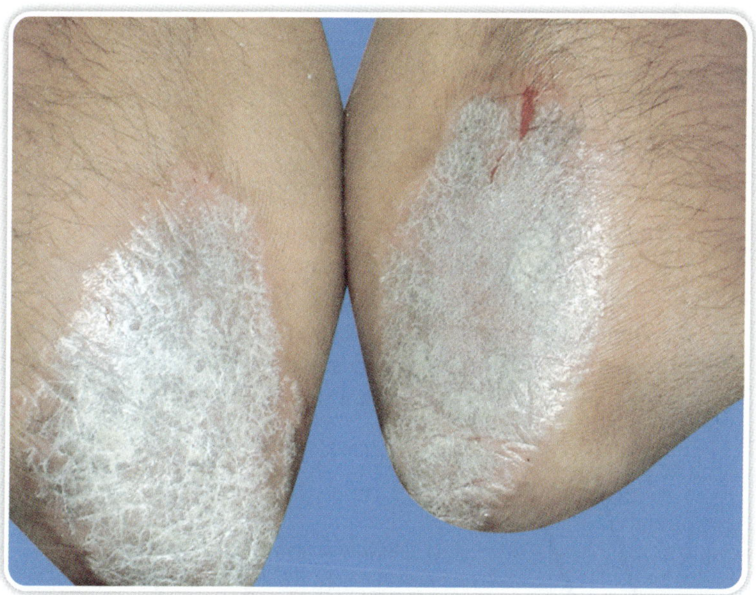

Fig. 3.1: Psoriasis: Well-defined erythematous plaques surmounted with silver scales.

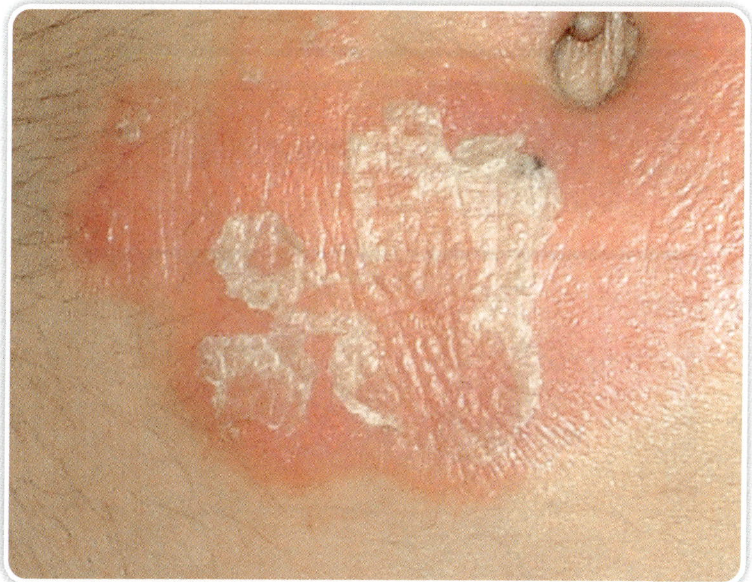

Fig. 3.2: Scales in psoriasis: Lamellar and nonadherent.

Auspitz Sign

Auspitz sign may help in the diagnosis of psoriasis.

- It helps to differentiate psoriasis from other skin conditions with morphologically similar lesions:
    - However, it is not positive in inverse psoriasis or pustular psoriasis.
    - On scalp lesions, even nonpsoriatic plaques, e.g., of seborrheic dermatitis may show a positive Auspitz sign.
- It is demonstrated in three steps **(Fig. 3.3)**:
    i. When the psoriatic plaque is scraped with a glass slide, the scales are accentuated and separate from the plaque, as silvery flakes (due to hyperkeratosis).

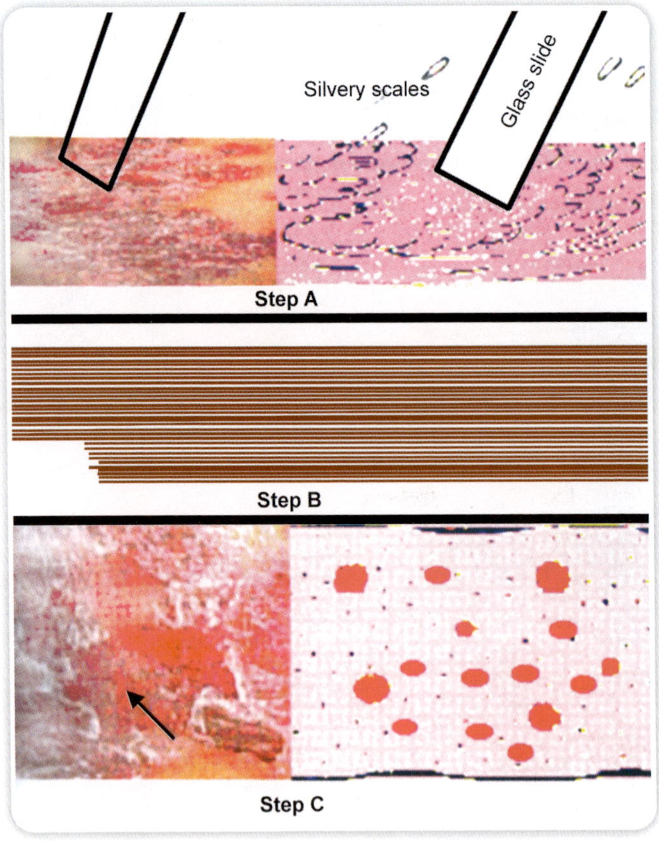

Fig. 3.3: Auspitz sign in psoriasis: In three steps.

ii. A thin glazed membrane appears, which is removable in toto on further scraping.

iii. Within a few seconds of mechanical removal of the membrane, pinpoint droplets of blood appear on the erythematous surface (due to dilated and tortuous blood vessels in papillary dermis).

Koebner's Phenomenon

Koebner's phenomenon or isomorphic phenomenon[1] is seen in approximately 38–76% of patients.

- It indicates actively spreading disease and is most frequently seen in patients with early-onset psoriasis.
- Lesions of psoriasis develop at sites of nonspecific trauma, e.g., cuts, surgical wounds, scratch marks, and even burns. Trauma-induced lesions are often linear **(Fig. 3.4)**.

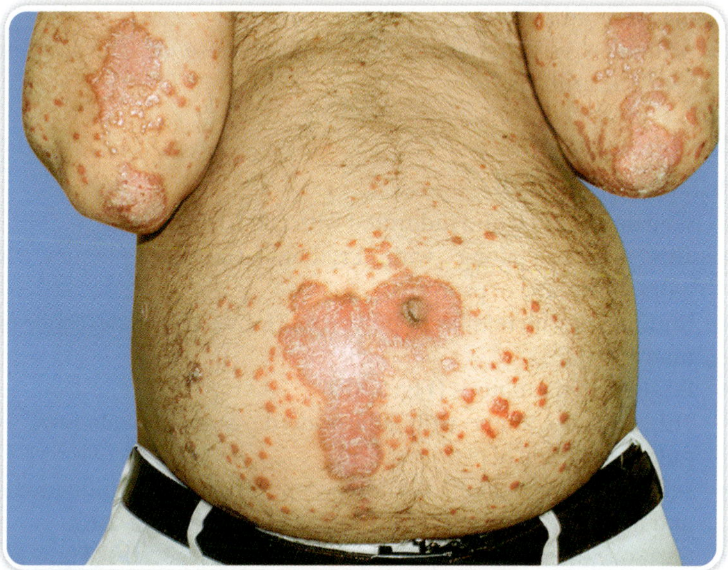

Fig. 3.4: Koebner's phenomenon: Psoriasis lesions developing at the site of surgical scar.

---

[1] The Koebner's phenomenon is a reaction where skin diseases such as psoriasis, lichen planus, and vitiligo can produce lesions at locations of skin injury. In contrast, the pseudo-isomorphic phenomenon refers to the appearance of lesions in conditions such as plane warts, molluscum contagiosum, and eczema at sites of previous damage.

- Clearing of existing psoriasis following injury has been observed and is termed as *reverse Koebner's phenomenon.*[2]

Patterns of Psoriasis

Chronic Plaque Psoriasis

Symptoms

- The chief complaint of patients with psoriasis is cosmetic unacceptability of skin lesions, resulting in lowered self-esteem and feeling of being an outcast socially.
- Pruritus is common, especially on scalp and anogenital psoriasis, though lesions may be asymptomatic.
- Pain may be present in lesions on palms and soles, especially if there is fissuring.
- Patients with generalized psoriasis may be intolerant to extremes of temperatures.
- Arthralgia is a frequent complaint, because of concomitant psoriatic arthritis.

Morphology

Plaques of psoriasis are:
- Well demarcated and indurated with clear-cut borders.
- This feature, along with erythema of the plaques, is pathognomonic of psoriasis.
- Borders may be regular or polycyclic (formed by coalescence of many plaques).
- Brightly erythematous **(Fig. 3.5)**.
- This feature, along with sharp demarcation of plaques, is pathognomonic of psoriasis.
- Brightness of erythema is less perceptible in darker individuals and in them, the lesions often appear lichenoid **(Fig. 3.6)**.
- Surmounted with noncoherent, lamellar silvery scales **(Fig. 3.2)**.
- If scaling is minimal, it can be accentuated by scraping the lesion with a glass slide *(Grattage test)*.
- Scales are minimal or absent in flexures.

---

[2] The reverse Koebner's phenomenon is when skin lesions improve following injury rather than worsen. It is less common and not fully understood.

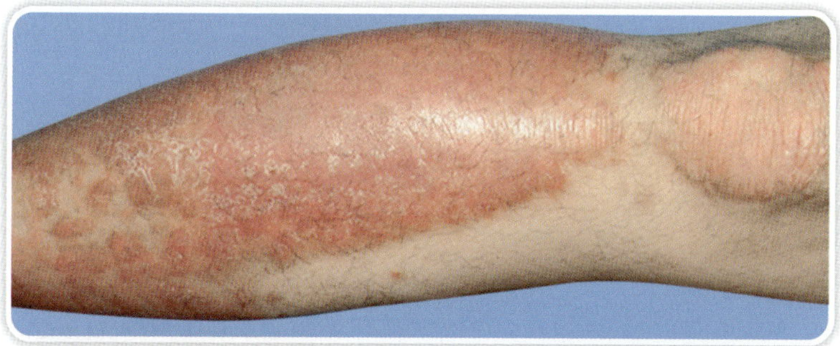

Fig. 3.5: Erythematous plaques: The erythema in psoriasis is typically bright.

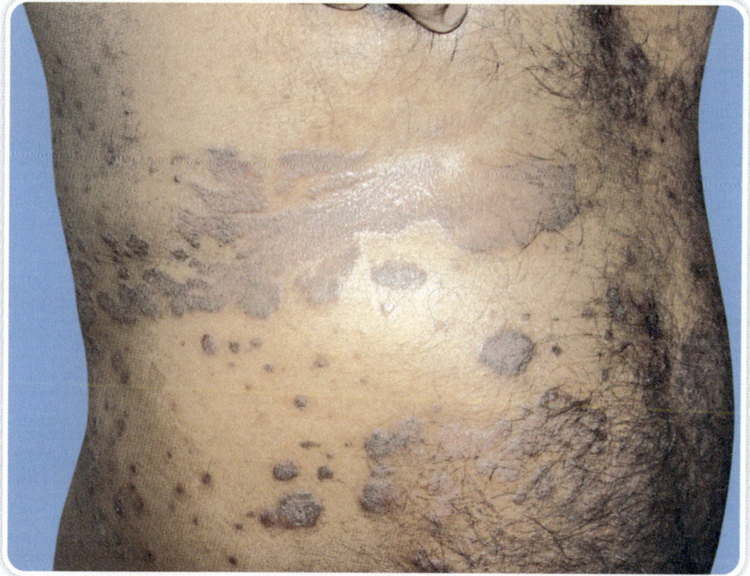

Fig. 3.6: Lichenoid lesions: Erythema is less perceptible in darker individuals and in them the lesions often appear lichenoid.

- Scales may be profuse and adherent on scalp as well as in elephantine psoriasis **(Fig. 3.7)**.
- Scales may be adherent and conical in Reiter's disease **(Fig. 3.8)**.
- Often surrounded by a ring of hypopigmentation, *ring of Woronoff*[3] **(Fig. 3.9)**.

---

[3] The "Ring of Woronoff" is an uncommon clinical sign in psoriasis, where a hypopigmented ring surrounds a psoriatic plaque. It indicates a zone of reduced inflammation.

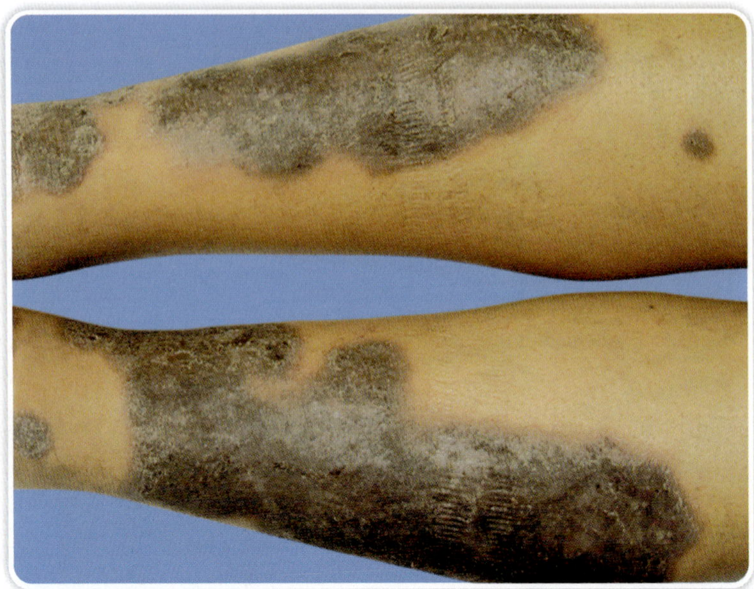

Fig. 3.7: Elephantine psoriasis: Large plaques with gross hyperkeratosis.

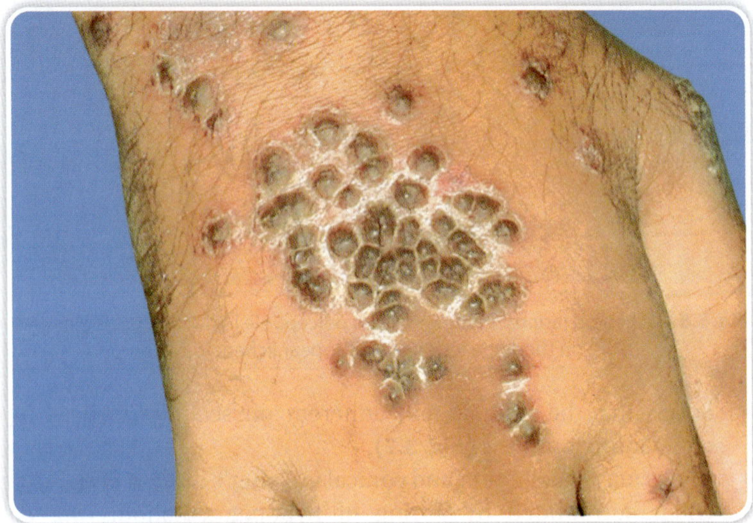

Fig. 3.8: Conical scales: As seen in rupioid psoriasis.

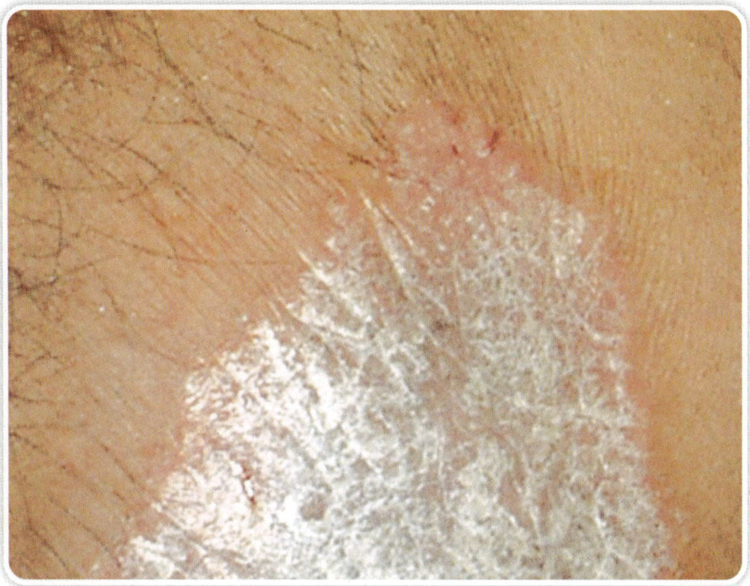

Fig. 3.9: Ring of Woronoff: Plaques of psoriasis are often surrounded by a ring of hypopigmentation.

- Positive Auspitz sign **(Fig. 3.3)**
- *Shape*: The shape of psoriatic plaques is variable:
  - Initial plaques are discoid.
  - As they enlarge, they coalesce to form polycyclic **(Fig. 3.10)** or arciform lesions *(psoriasis gyrata)*.
  - Occasionally, there is partial central clearing **(Fig. 3.11)**, resulting in annular lesions *(annular psoriasis)*.
  - Sometimes the lesions are linear[4] **(Fig. 3.12)**, geographic, or serpiginous.
- *Size*: It varies from small to large plaques, which may cover large areas of the trunk.

---

[4] *Linear lesions*: Such lesions should be differentiated from psoriasiform inflammatory linear epidermal nevus and nevoid psoriasis.

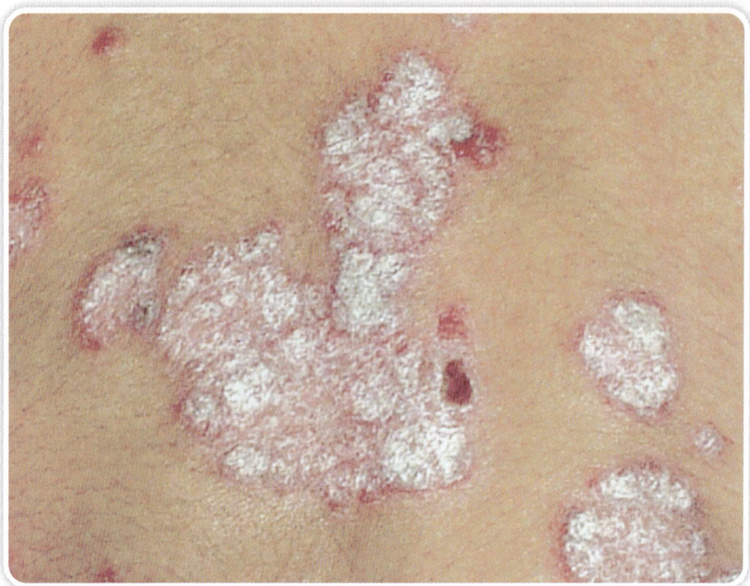

Fig. 3.10: Polycyclic plaques: As plaques of psoriasis enlarge, they coalesce to form polycyclic lesions.

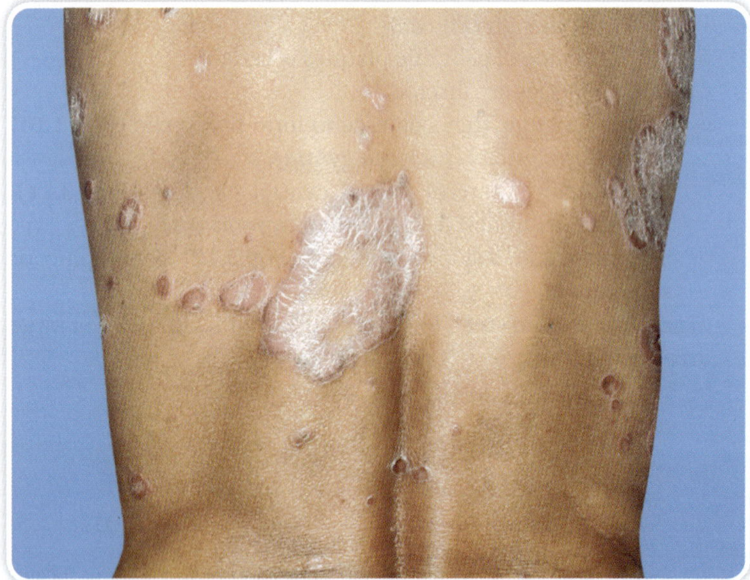

Fig. 3.11: Annular psoriasis: Partial central clearing results in annular plaques.

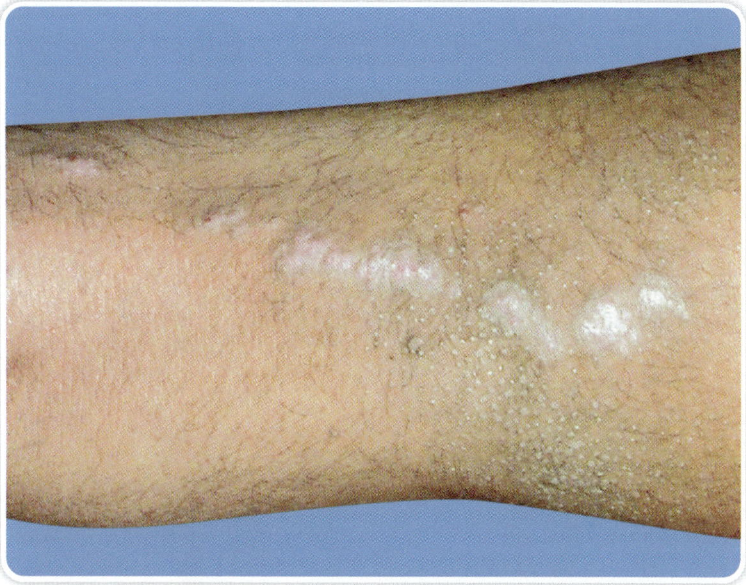

Fig. 3.12: Linear lesions: Erythematous scaly linear plaques. Such lesions should be differentiated from psoriasiform inflammatory linear verrucous epidermal nevus and nevoid psoriasis.

Sites of Predilection

- Lesions may be localized to one or more sites of predilection **(Fig. 3.13)**: Elbows, knees, sacral and gluteal region, scalp, palms and soles, and umbilicus. Or may occur anywhere on the body.
- Photo-exposed areas are usually spared. Face is uncommonly involved and its involvement usually indicates refractory type of psoriasis. However, in some patients, the lesions may be predominantly in photo-exposed areas **(Fig. 3.14)**. In such patients, phototherapy may aggravate the lesions and patients may have summer exacerbation.
- In inverse psoriasis, lesions are localized to axillae, groins, perianal, and inframammary regions, and neck.

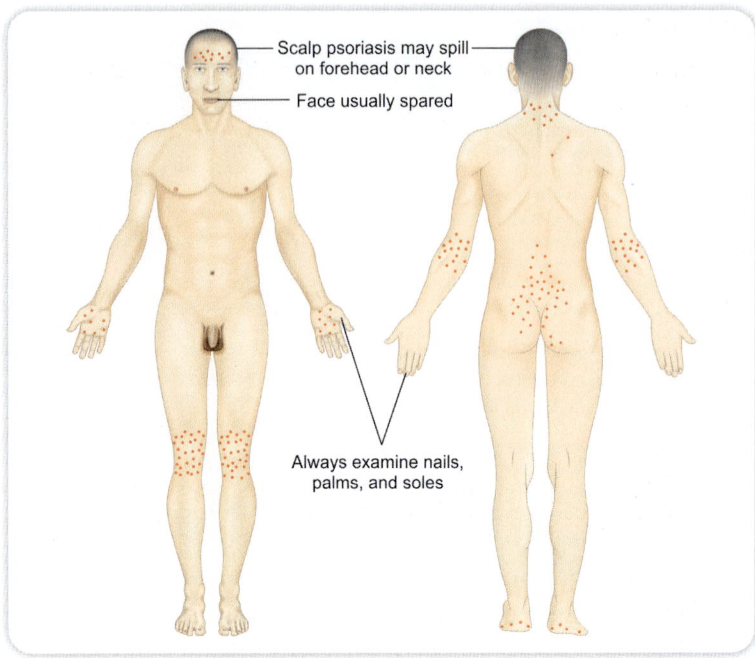

Fig. 3.13: Sites of predilection.

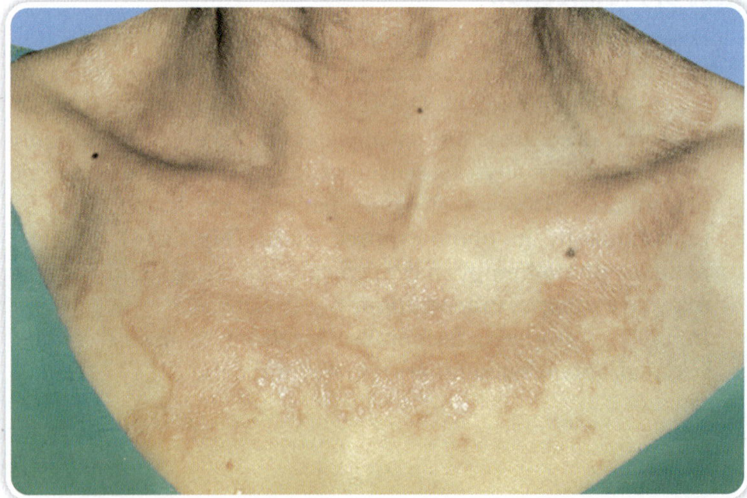

Fig. 3.14: Psoriasis in photo-exposed sites: In such patients, the plaques are present on face, nape and V of neck, and dorsolateral aspects of forearms (and waist in sari-wearing women).

Distribution

- Sometimes only a single site is involved (like scalp or palms and soles).
- Often multiple sites are involved; then it usually has a bilateral, often symmetrical distribution.
- Occasionally, lesions are generalized.

Variants

Palmar and Plantar Psoriasis

- *Involvement of palms and soles may either be*:
  - Part of generalized psoriasis.
  - Or as the only site involved.
- *Lesions are*:
  - Well demarcated, erythematous plaques **(Fig. 3.15)**. Sometimes, the involvement is diffuse **(Fig. 3.16)**.

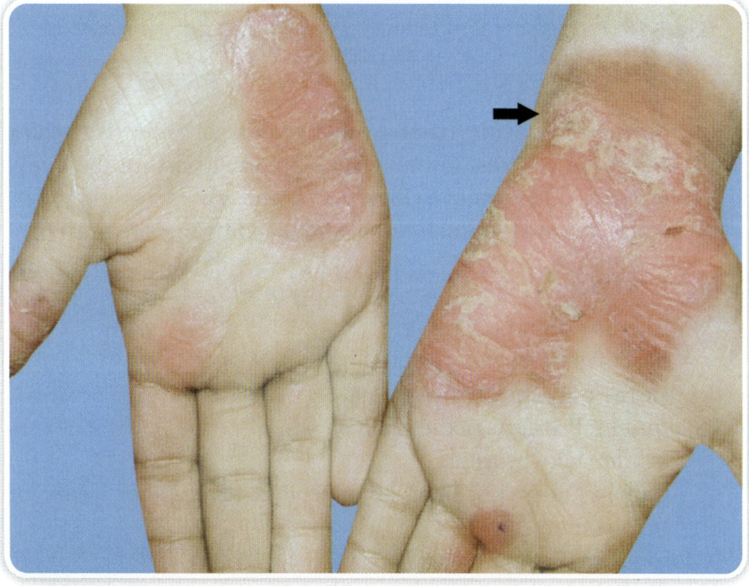

Fig. 3.15: Psoriasis of palms: Well-demarcated, erythematous scaly plaques. Note spillage on the wrist.

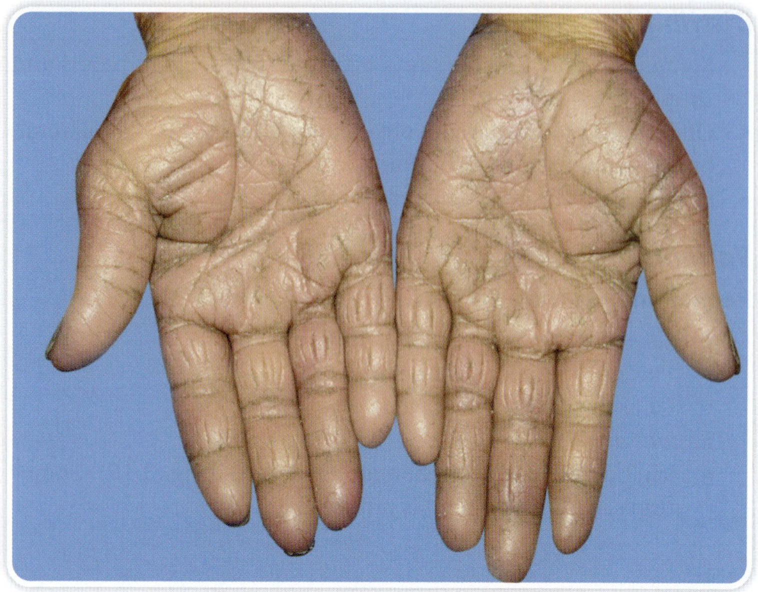

Fig. 3.16: Psoriasis of palms: Diffuse yet well-demarcated, erythematous scaly plaque.

- ○ Surmounted with massive silvery white or yellowish scales which, in contrast to the lesions on other parts of the body, are difficult to remove **(Figs. 3.17A and B)**.
- ○ Cracking and painful fissures and bleeding may be present.

Scalp Psoriasis

- *Scalp psoriasis may either be*:
  - ○ Part of generalized psoriasis.
  - ○ Or the only site involved.
- *Symptoms*: Psoriasis of the scalp:
  - ○ Is often very pruritic.
  - ○ Usually does not lead to hair loss, even after years of involvement.
- *Morphology*: Scalp lesions are:
  - ○ Sharply marginated, often with thick adherent scales. If the scales are asbestos-like and firmly adherent to scalp and hair, the condition is labeled as *pityriasis amiantacea* **(Fig. 3.18)**.
  - ○ Either scattered and discrete. Or the entire scalp may be diffusely involved, often spilling onto forehead **(Fig. 3.19)** and nape of neck.

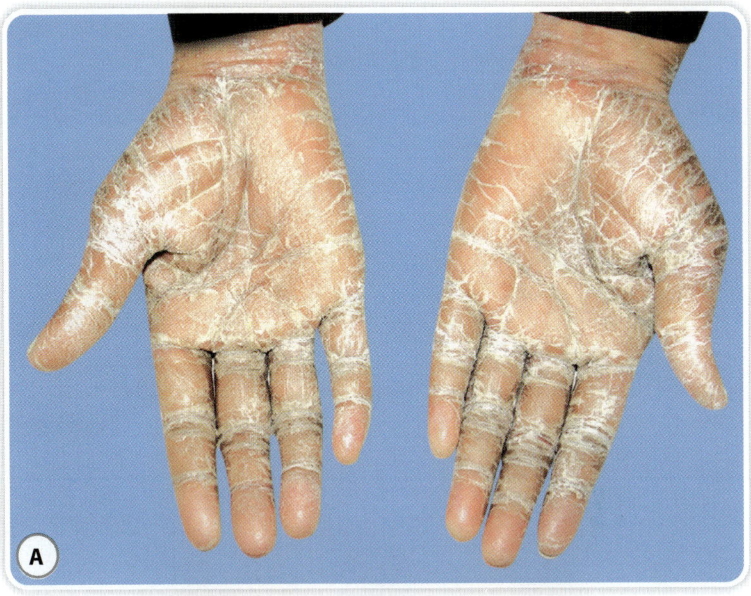

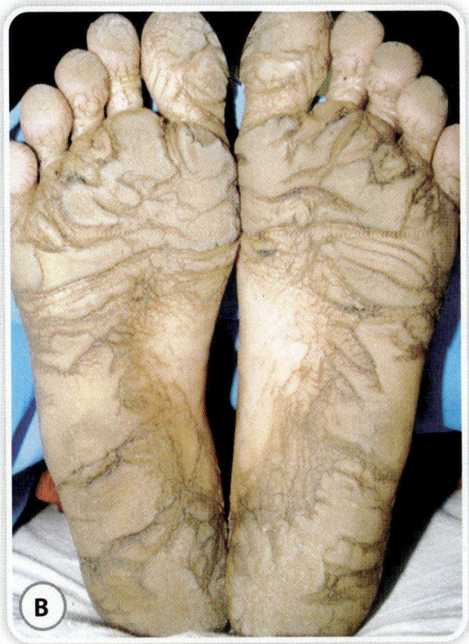

Figs. 3.17A and B: Psoriasis of palms and soles: Diffuse scaly plaques. Unlike on other parts, scales in psoriasis of palms and soles are often adherent.

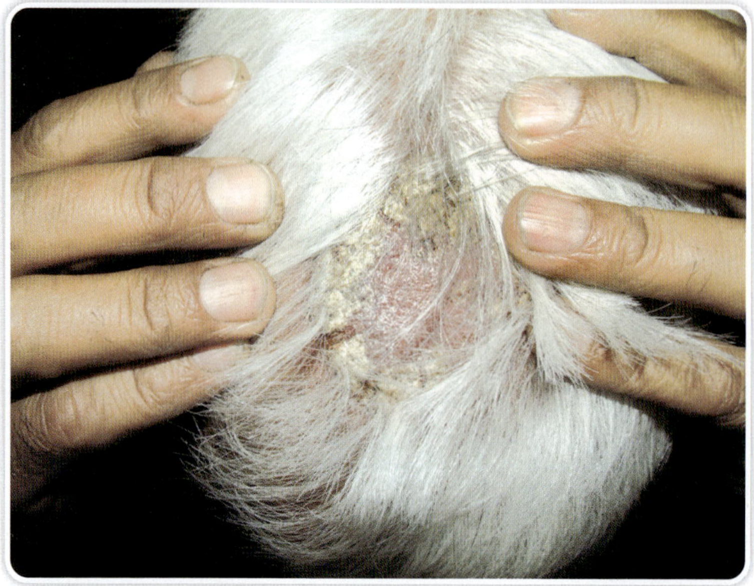

Fig. 3.18: Psoriasis of scalp: Plaque with thick adherent scales, pityriasis amiantacea.

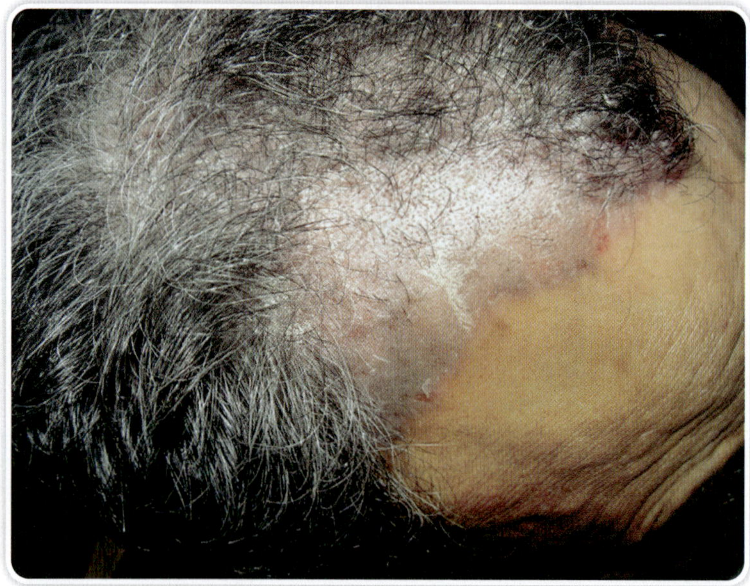

Fig. 3.19: Psoriasis of scalp: Well-defined erythematous scaly plaque spilling on to the forehead.

Inverse Psoriasis (Flexural Psoriasis)

- Flexural lesions can be a part of generalized psoriasis. In some patients, all lesions may exclusively be flexural.
- *Morphology*: Due to the moistness of sites, psoriatic plaques are usually not scaly but are bright red (so called *pinking*) and may be fissured **(Fig. 3.20)**.
- *Sites*: Axillae, groins **(Fig. 3.21)**, perianal region, inframammary region, prenatal cleft, and neck.
- In the absence of scaling, sharp demarcation and bright erythema help to differentiate inverse psoriasis from intertrigo, candidiasis, contact dermatitis, and tinea cruris.

Acute Guttate Psoriasis

Guttate: Latin *gutta,* meaning "drop".

Age

Acute guttate psoriasis is seen in children, adolescent, and young adults.

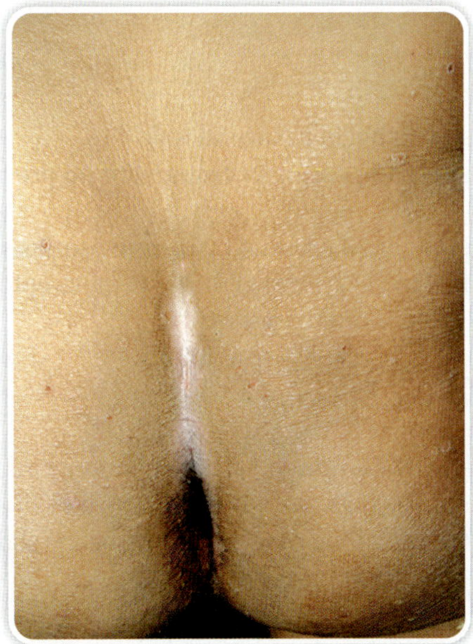

Fig. 3.20: Inverse psoriasis: Well-demarcated, erythematous plaques (so-called "pinking") of the intergluteal fold.

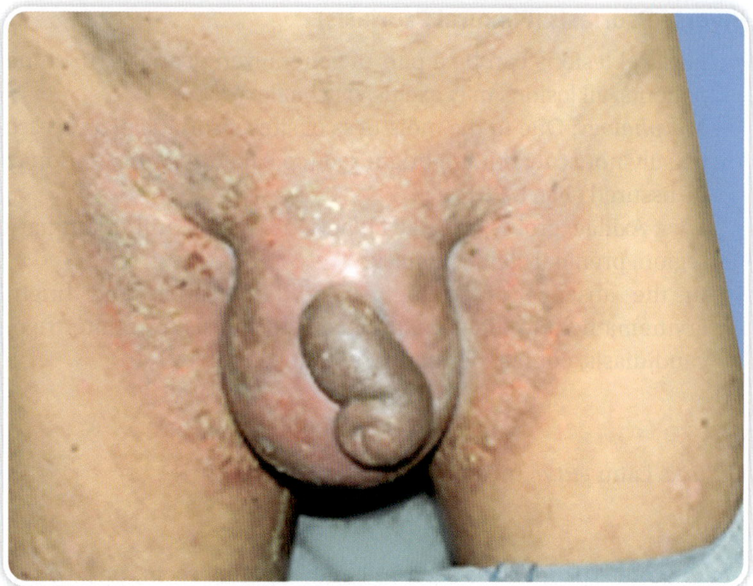

Fig. 3.21: Inverse psoriasis: Well-demarcated, erythematous plaques with minimal scaling in the groins. This patient also had pustular lesions.

Onset

Guttate psoriasis can begin in several ways:

- Eruptive lesions, appearing in crops, with no previous history of psoriasis.
- Acute exacerbation of preexisting plaque psoriasis.

A preceding (by 1–2 weeks) history of streptococcal upper respiratory infection is often present.

Morphology

- Lesions are discrete and scattered.
- Drop-like, small (2.0 mm to 1.0 cm), salmon-pink papules, with or without scales **(Figs. 3.22 and 3.23)**. Scales, if absent, can be accentuated by scraping the lesion with a glass slide.

Sites of Predilection

- Generally, concentrated on the trunk
- Fewer lesions on the face and scalp
- Spares palms and soles

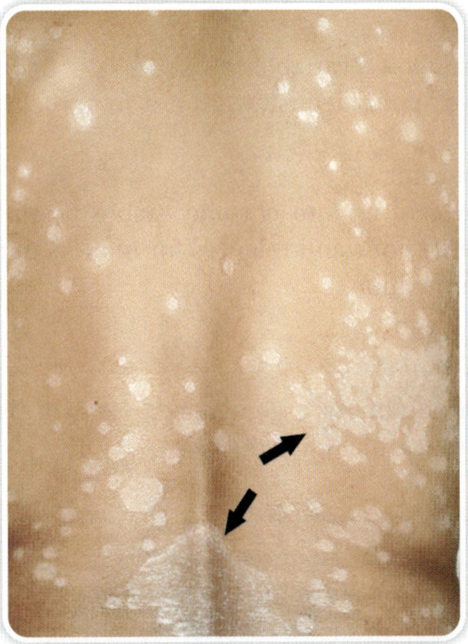

Fig. 3.22: Guttate psoriasis: Drop-like small pink papules with easily removable scales, present on the trunk. Note that in this patient, guttate lesions erupted in a person with chronic plaque psoriasis.

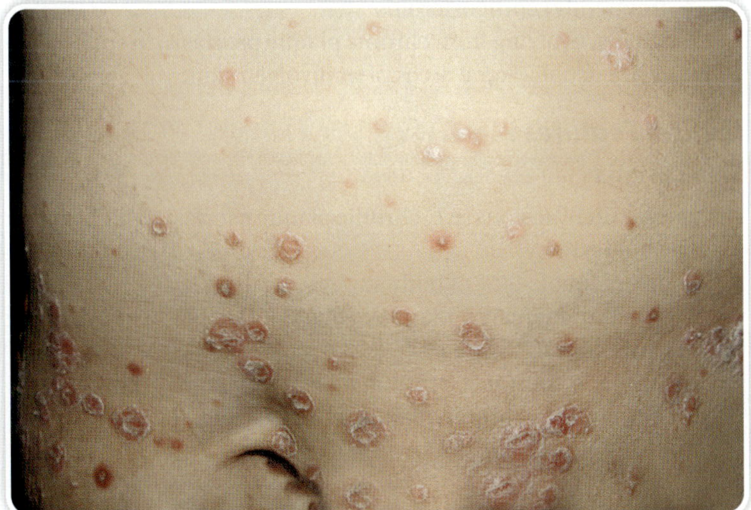

Fig. 3.23: Guttate psoriasis: Drop-like small pink papules with easily removable scales, present on the trunk.

Course

Guttate lesions follow a variable course:

- May resolve spontaneously within a few weeks, even without treatment.
- May be recurrent.
- More often evolves into chronic, stable psoriasis which may undergo remissions and relapses for months or years and be a life-long companion.

Psoriatic Erythroderma

Psoriatic erythroderma is a generalized form of psoriasis, which affects all body sites, including the face.

Onset

Psoriatic erythroderma can develop:

- Suddenly, as a generalized erythema with little or no areas of uninvolved skin. In such a case, it may develop due to:
  - Intolerance to treatment, e.g., anthralin, ultraviolet B (UVB), and even coal tar preparations, representing a generalized Koebner's phenomenon.
  - Withdrawal of systemic (more frequently) or topical (less frequently) corticosteroids.
- Gradually, evolving from chronic plaque psoriasis; in such a case there are usually some areas of uninvolved skin.

Clinical Features

Skin Lesions

- Severely itchy lesions (*c.f.,* chronic plaque psoriasis which may or may not be itchy).
- Involvement of >90% of body surface.
- Less well-demarcated plaques **(Fig. 3.24)** or diffuse erythema with exfoliation.
- Erythema is the most prominent feature. Scaling may be less as compared to chronic plaque psoriasis **(Fig. 3.25)** or may be profuse.

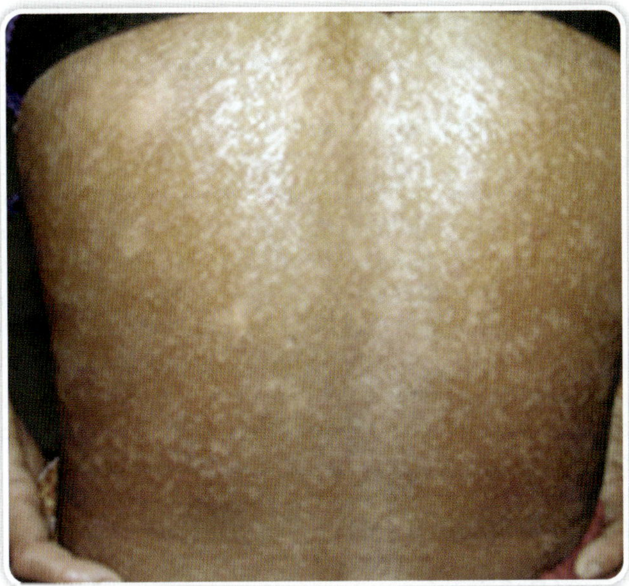

Fig. 3.24: Psoriatic erythroderma: Plaques of psoriasis begin to lose their margin and become generalized.

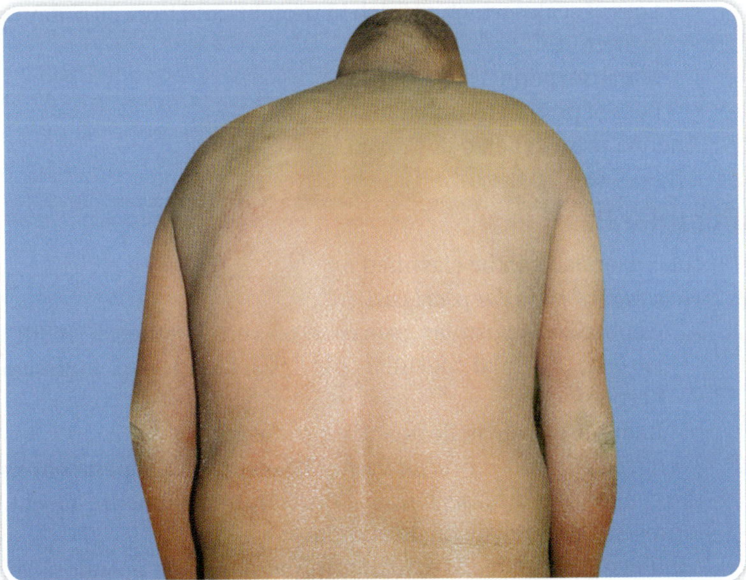

Fig. 3.25: Psoriatic erythroderma: Generalized erythema with minimal scaling.

Metabolic Changes

Persistent generalized erythema and scaling can have several metabolic effects:

- *Thermoregulation*: Temperature control is defective and erythroderma can lead to both:
  - Hyperthermia, in hot ambient temperatures (of tropics), because of hypohidrosis due to occlusion of sweat ducts.
  - Hypothermia, more common in normal environmental temperatures, because of increased loss of heat from the vasodilatation in the skin.
- *Circulatory failure*: It is due to increased skin blood flow, increased blood volume, and increased cardiac output. This particularly happens in the presence of anemia, hypertension, and myocardial compromise.
- *Dehydration*: It is due to fluid loss from skin.
- *Malabsorption*: It is due to dermatopathic enteropathy.

Nutritional Deficiencies

The nutritional deficiencies which develop in psoriasis include:

- *Hypoproteinemia due to*:
  - Loss of scales which are rich in proteins and iron. 30 g/day of protein
  - Malabsorption
  - Loss of protein into skin tissue
- Anemia (iron deficiency/mixed)

Pustular Psoriasis

Pustular psoriasis can be classified as:

- *Generalized pustular psoriasis*:
  - Generalized pustular psoriasis of von Zumbusch (GPP), *variant*: Annular pustular psoriasis (APP) and impetigo herpetiformis
  - Infantile and juvenile pustular psoriasis
- *Localized pustular psoriasis*: It must be considered separate from the generalized disease, because systemic symptoms are absent. It presents as three distinct conditions:
  - i. Pustulosis palmaris et plantaris (palmoplantar pustulosis)
  - ii. Acrodermatitis continua of Hallopeau
  - iii. Psoriasis with pustules

Generalized Pustular Psoriasis of von Zumbusch

Generalized pustular psoriasis of von Zumbusch is a life-threatening medical problem with an abrupt onset and requiring aggressive therapy. The skin involvement is distinctive and is associated with constitutional symptoms. The patient may or may not have had a stable plaque psoriasis in the past.

Epidemiology

- Rare
- Occurs in adults, rarely in children

Pathogenesis

Unknown. A strong correlation exists between GPP and human leukocyte antigen (HLA-B27). The fever and leukocytosis which develop are due to the release of cytokines and chemokines from the skin into the circulation.

Precipitating Factors

- *Drugs (Table 2.1, page 4)*: Most important is withdrawal of steroids (more frequently systemic, less frequently topical).
- Infections
- Hypocalcemia
- Pregnancy

Onset of Lesions

The constellation of fiery-red erythema followed by pustules accompanied by fever occurs acutely, over a period of less than a day. As one crop of pustules dries, another wave appears, invariably accompanied by fever.

Symptoms

- *Cutaneous symptoms*: Marked burning and tenderness
- *Constitutional symptoms*: Headache, chills, fever, marked fatigue, and malaise

Skin Lesions

- *Morphology*:
  - Fiery red erythema (initially patchy, soon becoming confluent and generalized) appears suddenly. Within a few hours, a cluster of tiny, nonfollicular, very superficial creamy white pustules develop. The pustules either become confluent,

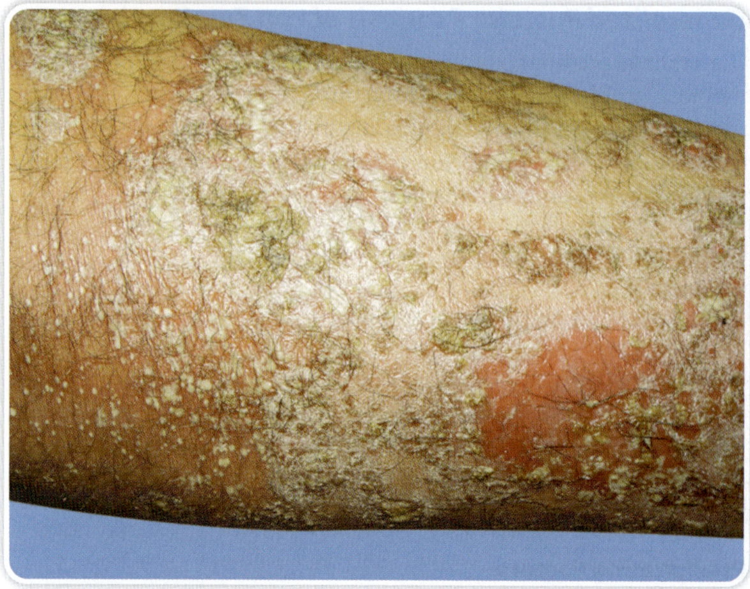

Fig. 3.26: Generalized acute pustular psoriasis (von Zumbusch): Multiple, creamy-white pustules on a fiery red base. Many areas show denudation, because pustules are literally wiped off (because they are superficial) resulting in red-oozing erosions.

forming circinate lesions and lakes of pus **(Fig. 3.26)** or are literally wiped off (because they are superficial), resulting in red-oozing erosions.

- ○ Lesions crust and as the crusts are shed, new crops of pustules may appear at the same site. Characteristically, new pustules appear in waves, usually accompanied by fever.
- ○ Nikolsky's sign may be positive in the untreated patient.
- *Sites of predilection*:
  - ○ The pustules are disseminated over the trunk and extremities, including the nail beds, palms, and soles.
  - ○ Face is usually spared, as seen with other forms of psoriasis.
- *Nails*:
  - ○ Nails are thickened and show onycholysis.
  - ○ Subungual "lakes of pus" **(Fig. 3.27)** may lead to shedding off of nails (anonychia).
  - ○ In patients with prolonged disease, fingertips may become atrophic.

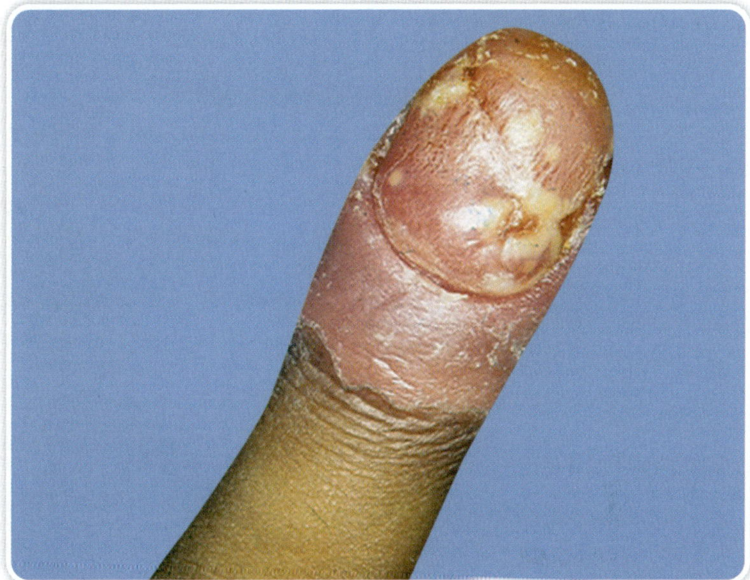

Fig. 3.27: Nails in pustular psoriasis: Characterized by subungual lakes of pus and onycholysis.

- *Hair:*
    - Hair loss (telogen effluvium) may develop in 2 or 3 months.
    - Gross hair loss occurs if lesions are present on scalp.
- *Mucous membranes:*
    - GPP is the only form of psoriasis that involves mucous membranes.
    - Circinate desquamation of the tongue resembling geographic tongue may develop **(Fig. 3.28)**.
- *Systemic features:*
    - Patient toxic
    - Tachycardia and tachypnea
    - Fever, often high grade
- *Complications:*
    - Hypoalbuminemia, due to loss of plasma proteins into tissues
    - Hypocalcemia
    - Oligemia can result in acute and fatal renal tubular necrosis, if not corrected.

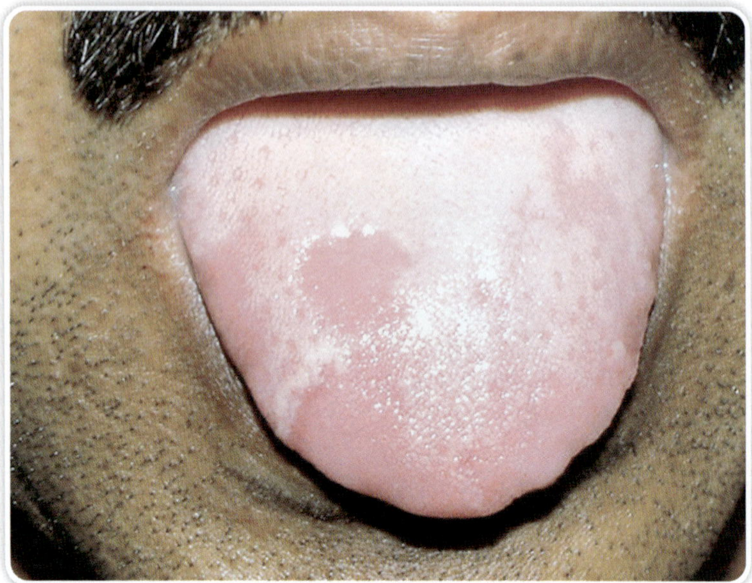

Fig. 3.28: Tongue in pustular psoriasis: Circinate desquamation of the tongue resembling geographic tongue.

- *Variants*:
  - APP:
    - Rare variant of pustular psoriasis, usually seen in children. Generally associated with fewer constitutional symptoms.
    - *Onset*: Lesions of APP usually appear either at the onset of GPP or during the course of GPP.
    - *Morphology*: The typical lesion of APP is an annular erythematous plaque, surmounted with pustules. The plaque enlarges to form large rings **(Fig. 3.29)**, often resembling lesions of erythema annular centrifugum.
- *Impetigo herpetiformis*:
  - Is von Zumbusch pustular psoriasis in pregnant women, usually in the last trimester. Often recurs in subsequent pregnancies.
  - Lesions are similar to those of APP **(Fig. 3.30)** and begin from inguinogenital region and other flexures.
  - Associated with constitutional symptoms and sometimes with hypocalcemia, leading to tetanic seizures.

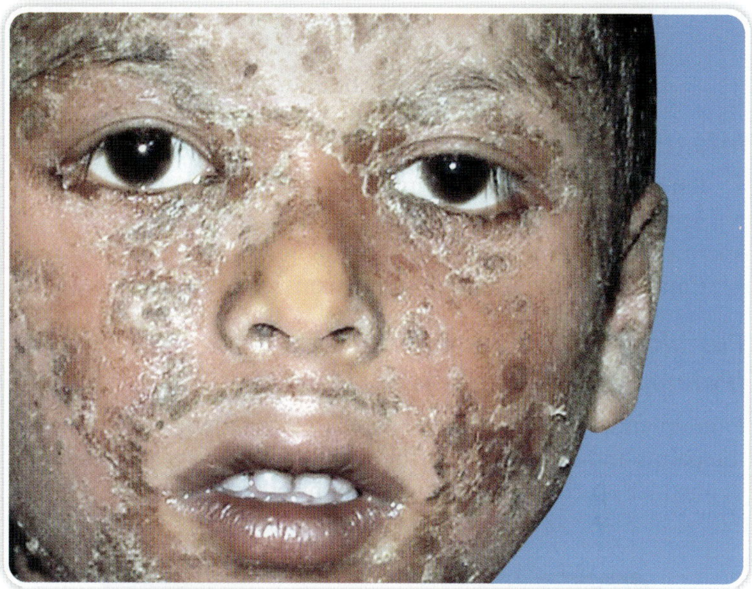

Fig. 3.29: Annular pustular psoriasis: Annular erythematous plaques surmounted with pustules in a child. The plaque enlarges to form large rings.

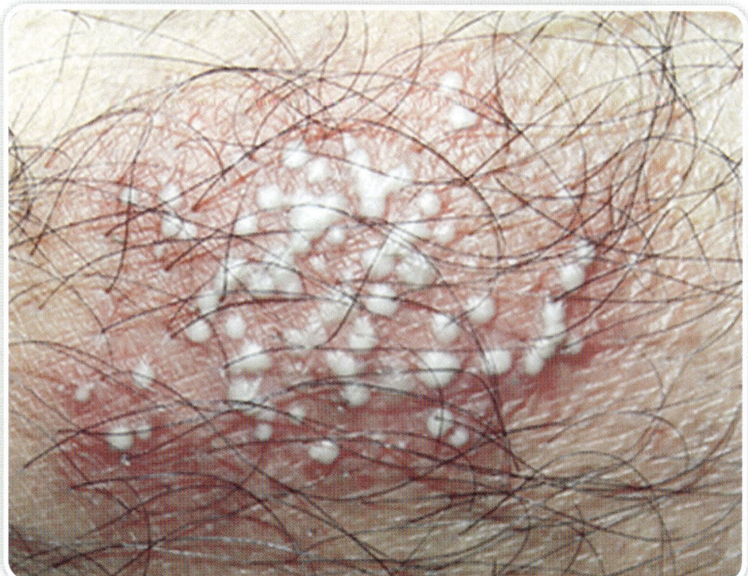

Fig. 3.30: Impetigo herpetiformis: Multiple, creamy-white pustules on a fiery red plaque on the thighs of a pregnant woman.

- ○ May be associated with placental insufficiency and fetal wastage.
- ○ Inflammatory polyarthritis common.

Infantile and Juvenile Pustular Psoriasis

- Rare type, usually seen in infants
- Annular/circinate lesions common **(Fig. 3.31)**
- Runs a benign course
- Confused with seborrheic and napkin dermatitis

Pustulosis Palmaris et Plantaris (Palmoplantar Pustulosis)

Palmoplantar pustulosis is a chronic, relapsing eruption limited to the palms and soles. It is considered by some to be a localized form of pustular psoriasis (Barber type) and by others as a separate entity.

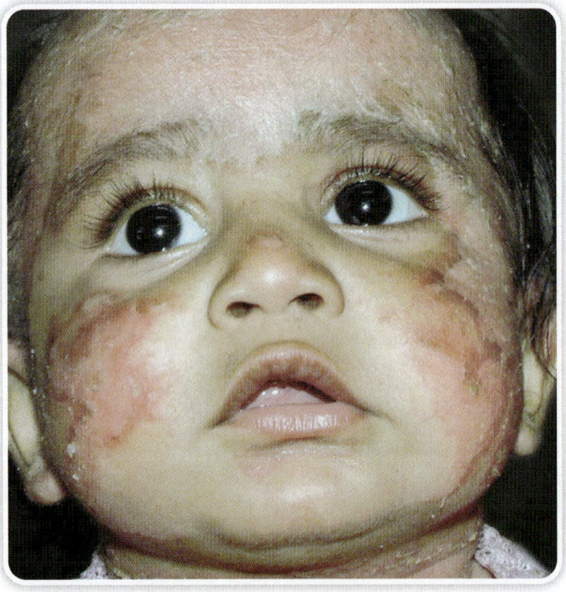

Fig. 3.31: Infantile and juvenile pustular psoriasis: Annular and circinate lesions in an infant.

Epidemiology

- *Incidence*: Less common than psoriasis vulgaris
- *Age of onset*: 50–60 years
- *Gender predilection*: Four times more common in females

Clinical Features

- *Symptoms*:
    - Stinging, burning, and itching
    - Eruption comes in waves
- *Morphology of lesions*: Pustules in various stages of evolution are typical:
    - Small (2–5 mm), deep-seated, creamy-yellow pustules, arise on a dusky-red, scaly background **(Fig. 3.32)** or on normal skin.
    - Evolve into crusts which finally exfoliate.

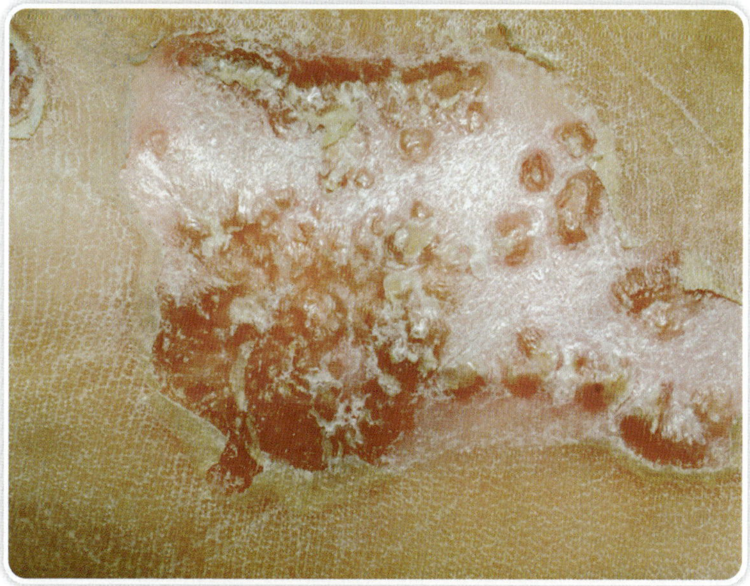

Fig. 3.32: Pustulosis palmaris et plantaris: Deep-seated, dusky-red, macules and creamy-yellow pustules progress to hyperkeratotic/crusted papules.

- *Sites of predilection*: Limited to palms and soles, appearing as either:
  - Single plaque
  - Multiple plaques, symmetrically involving both hands and feet. A predilection for thenar and hypothenar eminences (without extending proximal to the wrist line), flexoral aspects of fingers, heels, and insteps and sparing the acral portions of fingers and toes **(Fig. 3.33)**.
- *Course*: Persistent for years, characterized by unexplained remissions and exacerbations. Rarely, lesions of psoriasis vulgaris develop on other parts of body.
- *Associations*:
  - Hyper and hypothyroidism
  - Arthritis

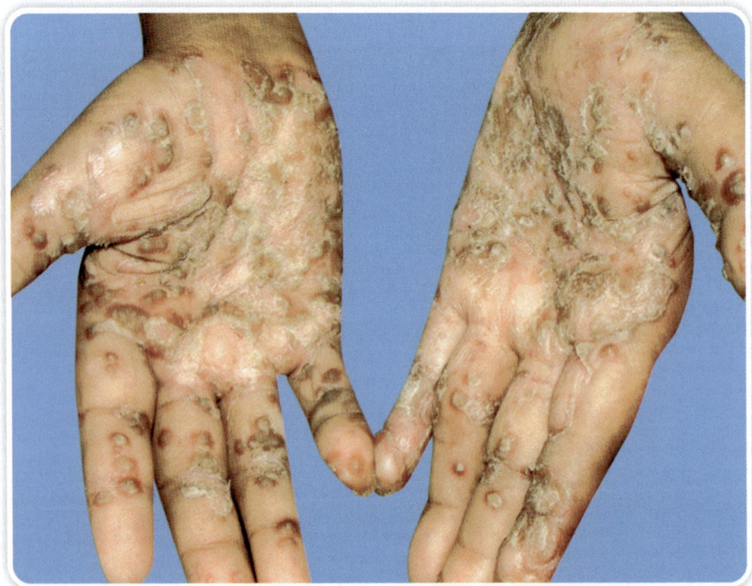

Fig. 3.33: Pustulosis palmaris et plantaris: Lesions are confined to the palms and/or soles without extending proximal to wrist. Note relative sparing of acral parts of digits.

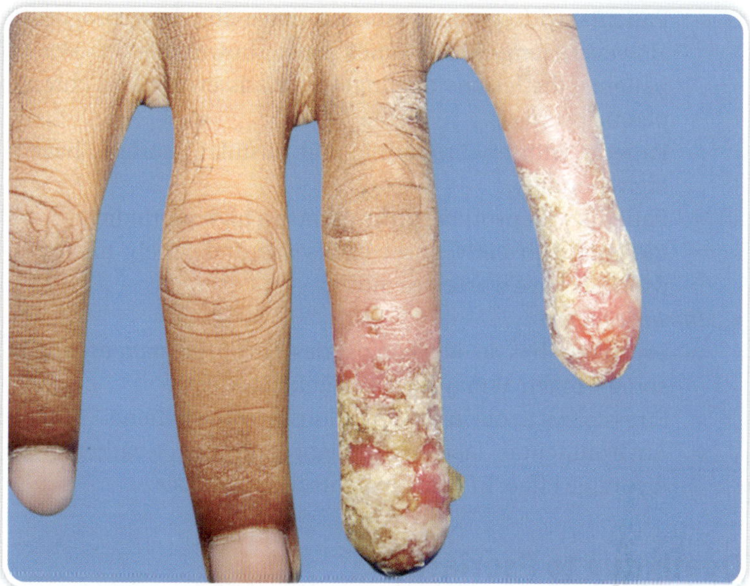

Fig. 3.34: Acrodermatitis continua of Hallopeau: Presents as chronic recurrent pustulation of nail folds, nail bed, and distal fingers leading to loss of nails.

Acrodermatitis Continua of Hallopeau

- This is a chronic recurrent pustulation of nail folds, nail bed, and distal fingers leading to loss of nails **(Fig. 3.34)**.
- It can occur in isolation or in association with pustular psoriasis of von Zumbusch.

Course of Psoriasis

Course and prognosis of psoriasis is uncertain, and it is not possible to predict the effect of any therapy in a patient, relapses being the rule, by whatever method the patient has been treated.

Several factors determine the course of psoriasis:

- *Type of psoriasis*:
  - Of the patients with chronic plaque psoriasis, 20–46% remit spontaneously without treatment for periods varying from 1 to 54 years, according to different studies.

- o Patients with guttate psoriasis have the best prognosis. However, long-term studies have shown that in 33% of patients, the lesions of guttate psoriasis evolve into chronic plaque psoriasis.
  - o Patients with erythrodermic and pustular psoriasis have a high mortality.
  - o Patients with psoriatic arthritis have a high morbidity.
  - o Patients with early onset of disease and family history of psoriasis have worse prognosis.
- *Intrinsic factors*:
  - o Pregnancy has no effect on psoriasis in 50% of patients and in some women, it may have a beneficial effect.
  - o Stress plays a role in exacerbations in some patients.
  - o Environmental factors: Sunlight and hot weather have favorable effect in many patients with psoriasis.

Death due to Psoriasis

Death due to psoriasis, though uncommon, can occur due to:
- *Erythroderma*: Due to temperature dysregulation, high output cardiac failure, and sepsis.
- *Generalized pustular psoriasis*: Due to hypocalcemia which may lead to tetany or cardiac complications.
- *Complications of arthritis*: Arthritis may make the patient bed ridden and prone to thrombosis and thromboembolism.
- *Side effects of drugs*: Rarely, a patient of psoriasis may succumb to the side effects of drugs (used for the treatment of severe psoriasis) like leukopenia, thrombocytopenia, and immunosuppression, leading to sepsis. Hepatic and renal damage are also known toxicities of antipsoriasis drugs.

Nail Changes

Introduction

In patients with psoriasis, nail changes are a common and significant manifestation, affecting both the quality of life and the functional ability of the patients. This chapter discusses the common nail changes seen in patients with psoriasis, ranging from minor pitting to severe onychodystrophy and anonychia. It provides a detailed look at the clinical features and underlying causes of these changes, helping in better diagnosis and management.

Epidemiology

- Nail changes are frequent (60%) in patients with psoriasis and are more common in patients with psoriatic arthritis.
- Finger nail involvement is seen in 50% of patients, while toe nail involvement is slightly less frequent (35%).
- Involvement is usually bilateral and often symmetrical.
- The nail changes range from minor defects of the nail plate (pits) to severe alterations of the plate (onychodystrophy) and loss of the nail plate (anonychia), depending on extent and duration of involvement of the nail organ **(Fig. 4.1)**.

Clinical Features

Pits

- Pits are the most common manifestation of nail psoriasis.
- These are formed due to defective keratinization (parakeratosis), the parakeratotic column on the dorsal surface of the nail plate falling off, to form a pit.

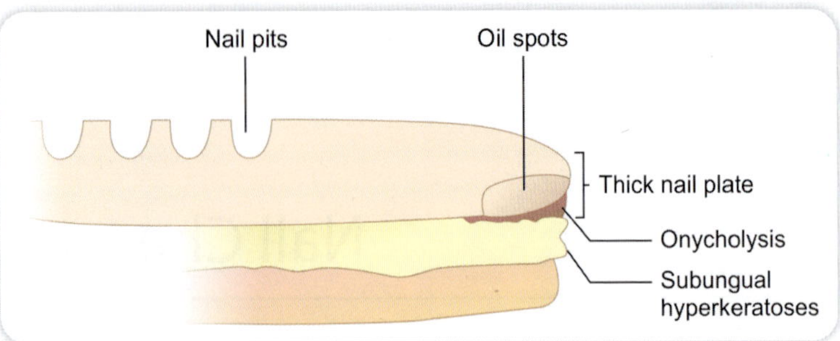

Fig. 4.1: Nails in psoriasis: Changes range from pits, thickening, and discoloration of nail plate, onycholysis, oil spots, and in severe cases loss of the nail plate (anonychia), depending on extent and duration of involvement of the nail organ.

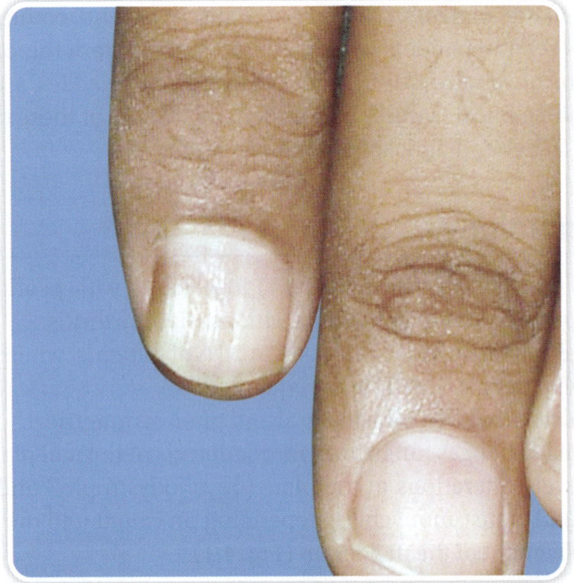

Fig. 4.2: Nail pits in psoriasis: May be arranged regularly in transverse/longitudinal rows resembling the surface of thimble. Or pits may be arranged haphazardly. They may be shallow or appear as large, punched out craters.

- These may be arranged regularly (in transverse/longitudinal rows resembling the surface of a thimble) or haphazardly. They may be shallow **(Fig. 4.2)** or deep like punched-out craters.

Oil Spot Sign

- Oil spot signs are almost pathognomonic of psoriasis.
- These are produced by focal parakeratosis of nail bed.
- These appear as yellowish-brown spots under the nail plate **(Fig. 4.3)**, which often extend distally toward the hyponychium.

Onycholysis

- Onycholysis is the separation of nail plate from nail bed.
- It results from extension of focal parakeratosis of the nail bed to the free edge of nail plate.
- It extends from proximal to distal edge but may also commence from the distal edge, leading to breach in the onychocorneal junction **(Fig. 4.4)**.
- It is aggravated by wet work.

Discoloration

- Major cause of the yellowish discoloration of nails is subungual hyperkeratosis and nail plate thickening.
- Superadded infection due to *Candida* and *Pseudomonas* species may impart a green color to the nail.

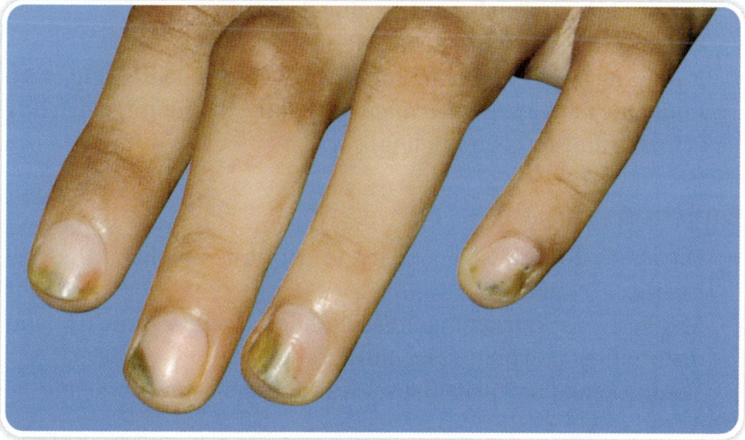

Fig. 4.3: Oil spot signs: Appear as yellowish-brown spots under the nail plate which often extend distally toward the hyponychium.

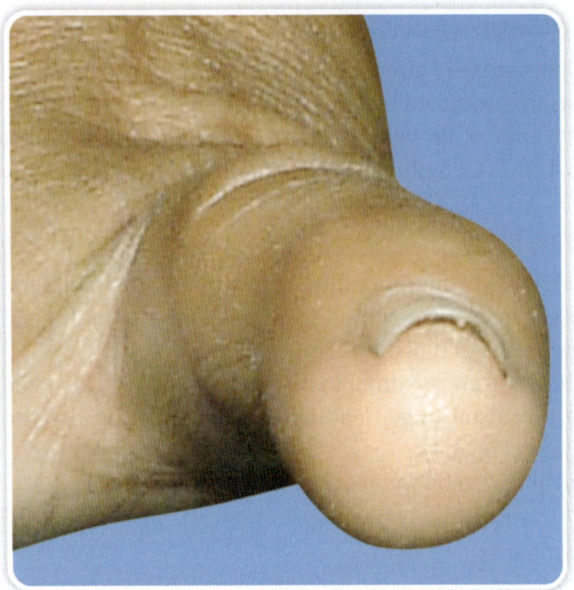

Fig. 4.4: Onycholysis: It is separation of nail plate from nail plate.

Subungual Hyperkeratosis

- Subungual hyperkeratosis represents nail bed hyperkeratosis.
- It extends both distally and proximally.
- When severe, can cause tenderness.
- It presents as accumulation of firm keratinous debris **(Fig. 4.5)**, under the nail (*c.f. in tinea unguium,* where the subungual debris is friable and shows tunneling).

Onychodystrophy

- Onychodystrophy is secondary to psoriasis involving the nail matrix.
- Manifests as thickening, discoloration (yellow brown), and distortion of nail plate **(Fig. 4.6)**.
- The thickened nail plate in psoriasis does not show tunneling.

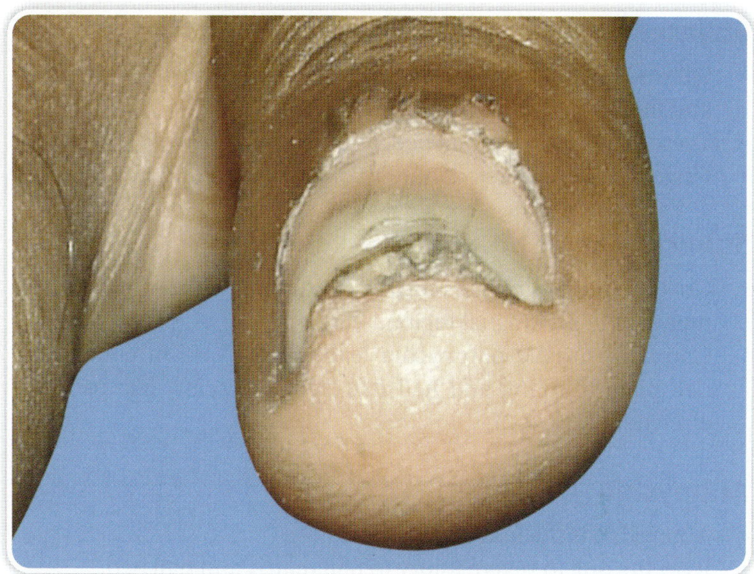

Fig. 4.5: Subungual hyperkeratosis: Presents as accumulation of firm keratinous debris under nail.

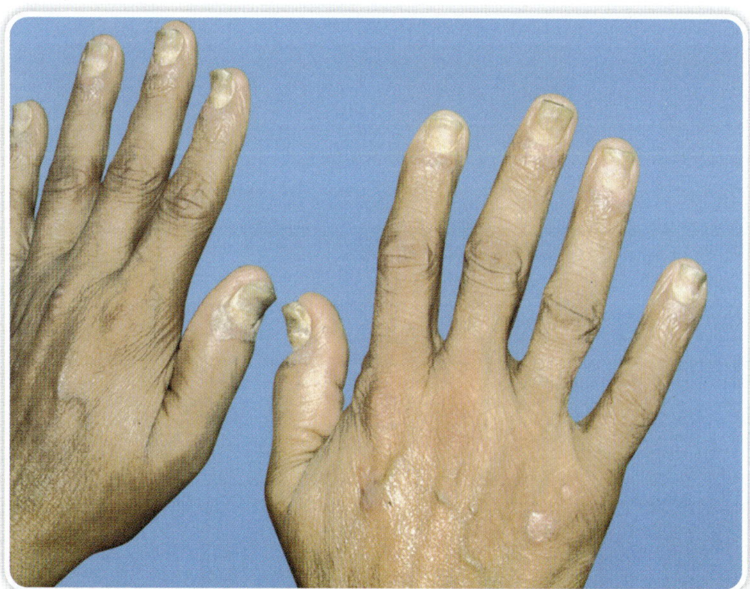

Fig. 4.6: Onychodystrophy: Manifests as thickening, discoloration (yellow-brown), and distortion of nail plate. The thickened nail plate in psoriasis is not friable and does not show tunneling.

Splinter Hemorrhages

- Splinter hemorrhages occur due to increased capillary tortuosity and their fragility in the nail bed.
- These are seen in the nail bed, as linear hemorrhagic bands.
- Finger nails are affected more than toe nails.

Subacute and Chronic Paronychia

- Gross disruption of nail matrix is associated with severe involvement of the periungual region.
- Chronic psoriatic paronychia leads to the loss of cuticle and nail plate thinning and nail fold becomes scaly, like psoriasis elsewhere **(Fig. 4.7)**.

Anonychia

- Anonychia is the loss of nail plate.
- It occurs due to severe injury to nail matrix and nail bed.
- It is typically seen in patients with generalized pustular psoriasis and acrodermatitis continua of Hallopeau **(Fig. 4.8)**.

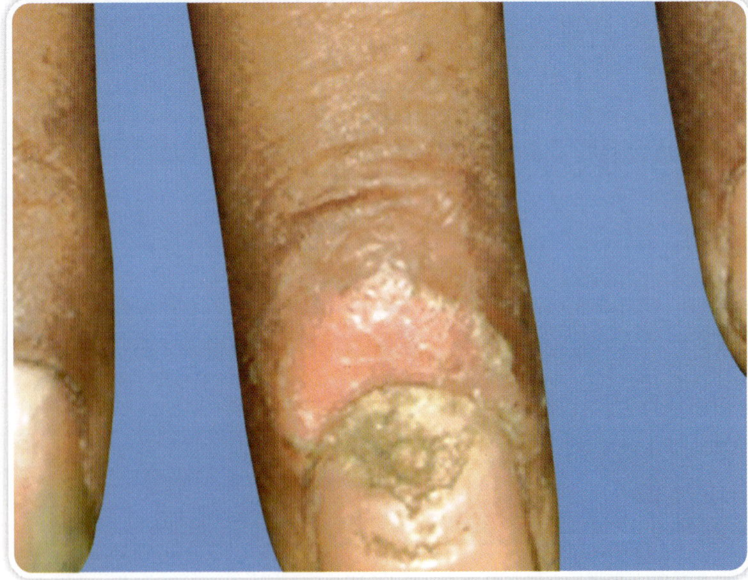

Fig. 4.7: Chronic psoriatic paronychia: Nail fold becomes scaly, like psoriasis elsewhere leading to loss of cuticle and thinning of nail plate.

Nail Changes in Pustular Psoriasis

- Nail involvement is frequent and severe in patients with generalized pustular psoriasis and acrodermatitis continua of Hallopeau. However, in palmoplantar pustulosis, nail changes are rare.
- *Manifestations depend on the acuteness and severity of involvement*:
    - In acute phase, characteristically subungual lakes of pus and onycholysis are seen.
    - As the disease subsides, the nail changes depend on severity of pustulation in acute phase:
        - If severe, it may lead to anonychia **(Fig. 4.8)**, which is shedding off of nail plate.
        - If less severe, onychodystrophy[1] and onycholysis develop.
- In patients with prolonged disease, fingertips may become atrophic.

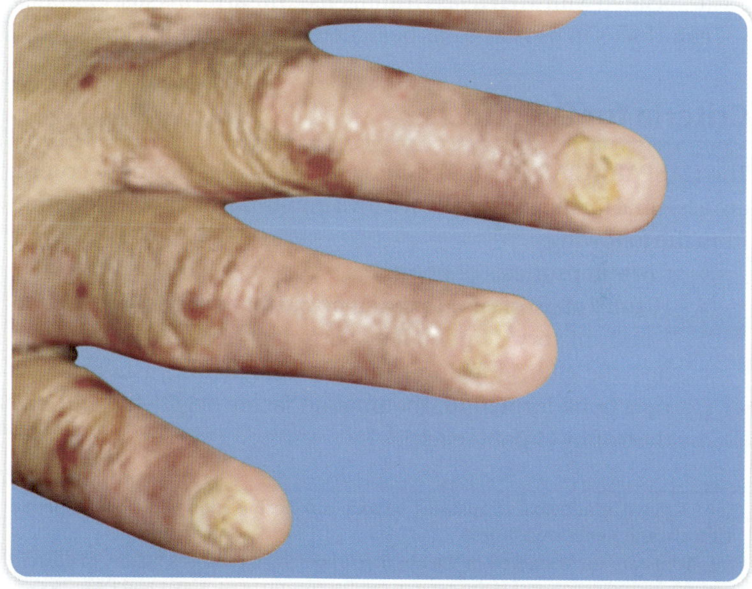

Fig. 4.8: Anonychia: Loss of nail plate due to severe injury to nail matrix, pustular psoriasis.

---

[1] *Onychodystrophy*: In the form of thickening, discoloration, and distortion of nail plate.

Arthritis

Introduction

- Psoriatic arthropathy (PsA) is a seronegative spondyloarthropathy[1] which is characterized by spondylitis and peripheral joint involvement of extremities, especially smaller joints.
- It is associated with major histocompatibility complex (MHC) class I antigens (in contrast to rheumatoid arthritis, which is associated with MHC class II antigens). The arthritis susceptibility gene locus in psoriasis has been detected on chromosome 16q.

Criteria for Diagnosis

The CASPAR (ClASsification criteria for Psoriatic ARthritis) criteria are essential for diagnosing PsA, with a minimum of 3 points required from the following:
- Current psoriasis (2 points)
- History of psoriasis (1 point if no current psoriasis)
- Family history[2] (1 point if no current or personal history)
- Specific clinical features including dactylitis, juxta-articular new bone formation, rheumatoid factor negativity, and nail dystrophy (1 point each).[3]

---

[1] Seronegative spondyloarthropathies include ankylosing spondylitis, enteropathic arthritis, and Reiter's syndrome.

[2] Family history is considered in the absence of personal psoriasis history or current symptoms and accounts for the genetic predisposition in psoriasis and PsA.

[3] Dactylitis refers to the swelling of fingers and toes resembling sausages, juxta-articular new bone formation indicates bone growth near joints, rheumatoid factor negativity helps differentiate PsA from rheumatoid arthritis, and nail dystrophy includes changes such as pitting, thickening, and onycholysis associated with psoriasis.

Epidemiology

- *Incidence*: A total of 2–7% of psoriasis patients have arthritis and the more severe the skin disease, more the chance of arthritis. Arthritis is more common with type 1 disease and may even precede skin lesions in 15–20% patients. In about 10% of patients with a diagnosis of PsA, skin lesions of psoriasis may never develop and in them, the diagnosis of PsA is made based on a positive family history of psoriasis.
- *Age*: Rare before 20 years of age.

Types

Five types of PsA are recognized:
1. Asymmetrical oligoarthritis
2. Distal interphalangeal arthritis
3. Symmetrical rheumatoid arthritis-like
4. Arthritis mutilans
5. Psoriatic spondylitis and sacroiliitis

Clinical Features

Asymmetrical Oligoarthritis

- Commonest (70%), but often overlooked.
- Involves only a few joints (sometimes only 1), asymmetrically.
- *Presentation*:
  - *Dactylitis*: Most frequent manifestation **(Fig. 5.1)**. Presents as sausage-shaped, tender swelling of 1 or more digits. Due to swelling and inflammation of flexor tendon sheaths or joint synovitis.
  - *Enthesitis*: It is swelling, redness, and tenderness at the site of insertion of the tendon (e.g., insertion of Achilles tendon on calcaneus).

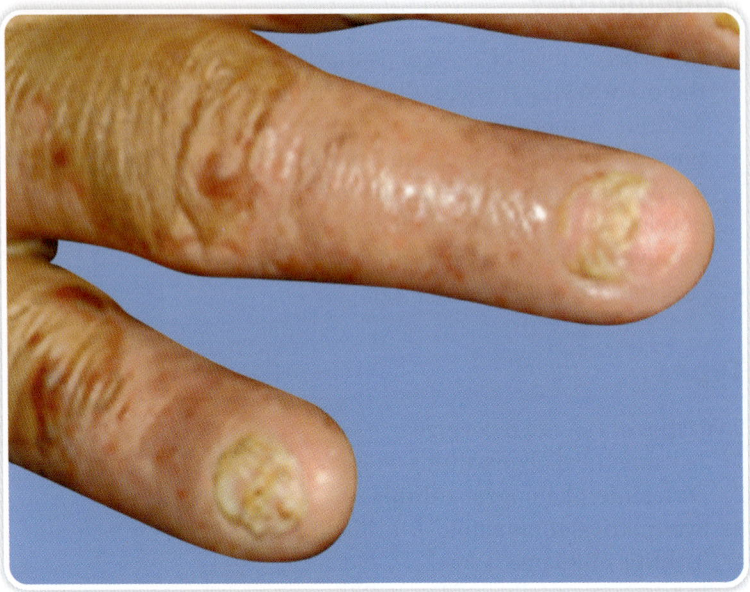

Fig. 5.1: Asymmetrical oligoarthritis presents most frequently as dactylitis which manifests as sausage shaped, tender swelling of 1 or more digits.

Distal Interphalangeal Arthritis

- Uncommon (5%)
- Asymmetrical involvement of a few distal interphalangeal joints of the hands and feet
- Psoriatic involvement of fingertips and periungual skin is frequently present **(Fig. 5.2)**. It may or may not be associated with psoriasis elsewhere.
- Usually associated with severe nail changes.

Symmetrical Rheumatoid Arthritis-like

- Seen in 15% of patients with psoriasis
- Symmetrical polyarthritis
- Resembles rheumatoid arthritis but differs from it:
  - By being seronegative
  - By being less severe
  - By being not associated with subcutaneous nodules

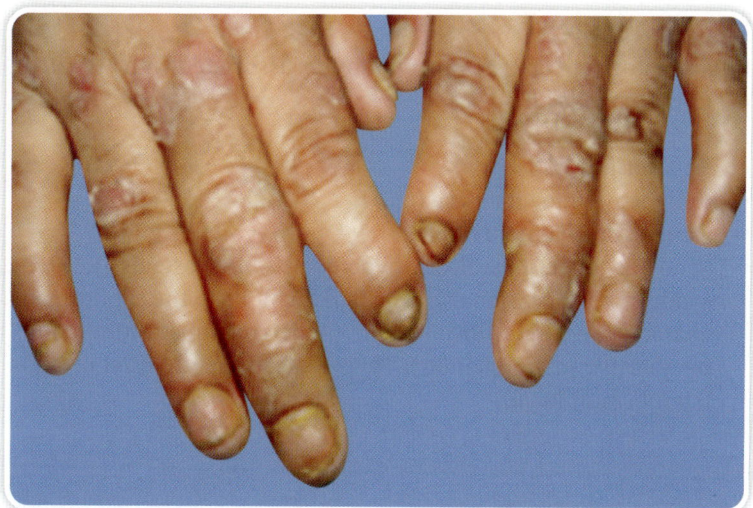

Fig. 5.2: Distal interphalangeal arthritis—asymmetrical involvement of a few distal interphalangeal joints of the hands and feet. Usually associated with nail changes.

Arthritis Mutilans

- Uncommon (5%)
- Severely deforming arthritis, involving fingers and toes, leading to digital shortening and ankylosis
- Radiologically bone erosions, gross osteolysis, and ankylosis are typical features.

Psoriatic Spondylitis and Sacroiliitis

- Though clinical axial involvement is seen in only 5% of patients, radiologically axial joints may be involved in up to 30% of psoriasis patients.
- Spinal involvement may be symptomatic or asymptomatic and may be associated with peripheral arthropathy.
- Three patterns of axial joint involvement are recognized:
    - Involvement of both spine and sacroiliac joints
    - Involvement of spine alone
    - Involvement of sacroiliac joints alone
- Less disabling than idiopathic spondylitis

Extra-articular Features

Inflammatory eye changes are commonly associated with arthritis:
- Conjunctivitis (20%)
- Uveitis (10%)
- Episcleritis (2%)
- Keratoconjunctivitis sicca (3%)
- Cardiac involvement rarely
- Synovitis, acne, pustulosis, hyperostosis, and osteitis (SAPHO) syndrome is occasionally associated with PsA. The syndrome is characterized by **s**ynovitis, **a**cne (acne conglobata/fulminans), **p**ustulosis (palmoplantar), **h**yperostosis, and **o**steomyelitis (sterile, multifocal).

Comorbidities

Introduction

Psoriasis is clearly linked with several behavioral and systemic comorbidities.

Metabolic Syndrome

- Metabolic syndrome **(Table 6.1)** is a combination of metabolic risk factors in an individual, including abdominal obesity, atherogenic dyslipidemia, elevated blood pressure, insulin resistance or glucose intolerance, prothrombotic state, and a proinflammatory state. Emerging evidence supports a strong link between psoriasis and metabolic syndrome, indicating a shared pathophysiological basis that emphasizes systemic inflammation. This relationship underlines the importance of a comprehensive assessment for metabolic syndrome in psoriasis patients.
- *Recommendations*: The primary goal of treating metabolic syndrome is to reduce cardiovascular disease. The American

TABLE 6.1: Components of metabolic syndrome.

Criteria	Measurement
- Elevated waist circumference	*Men*: >40 inch (102 cm); *Women*: >35 inch (88 cm)
- Elevated triglycerides	>150 mg/dL
- Reduced high-density lipoprotein (HDL) ("good") cholesterol	*Men*: <40 mg/dL
- Elevated blood pressure	>130/85 mm Hg
- Elevated fasting glucose	>100 mg/dL

TABLE 6.2: The American Heart Association (AHA) recommendations for the management of metabolic syndrome.	
Lifestyle	• *Diet*: Fruits, vegetables, whole grains, lean proteins; limit saturated fats, trans fats, sodium, added sugars • 150 minutes moderate or ≥75 minutes vigorous physical activity/week • Aim for 5–10% weight loss if overweight • Smoking cessation
Risk factor control	• *Blood pressure*: Target <130/80 mm Hg • *Lipids*: Adjust to lower low-density lipoprotein (LDL), triglycerides, and raise HDL • *Glucose*: Maintain <100 mg/dL
Pharmacotherapy and monitoring	• Medications as needed for blood pressure, lipids, and blood glucose • Regular monitoring of blood pressure, lipids, glucose

Heart Association recommends lifestyle modifications as a first-line therapy for metabolic syndrome **(Table 6.2)**.

Cardiovascular and Respiratory System

- Some studies have shown an increased risk of arterial and venous occlusive disease in patients with psoriasis.
- Patients with erythroderma and preexisting compromised cardiac function may occasionally experience high-output cardiac failure.
- Pulmonary fibrosis may rarely occur in patients with psoriatic arthropathy. This is more frequent in patients treated with methotrexate.
- Emerging evidence also associates psoriasis with an increased risk of chronic obstructive pulmonary disease (COPD).

Skin Cancer

- There is no apparent increase in skin cancer or internal malignancies in psoriatic patients compared to the general population.
- However, there may be an increase in nonmelanoma skin cancers in patients of psoriasis treated with phototherapy.

Liver

- There is no increased incidence of hepatic dysfunction in psoriasis.
- However, there are reports of increased susceptibility to hepatotoxic effects of methotrexate in patients with psoriasis.
- Furthermore, recent findings suggest a higher prevalence of nonalcoholic fatty liver disease (NAFLD) in psoriasis patients.

Kidney

- There is no increased incidence of renal changes in psoriasis.
- Infrequently, glomerulonephritis may be associated with post-streptococcal guttate psoriasis.
- In rare cases, renal amyloidosis may develop in patients with long-standing psoriatic arthropathy.

Ocular Changes

- A total of 10% of patients with psoriasis have ocular changes, including eyelid involvement.
- There is no increased incidence of cataract.
- Anterior uveitis and conjunctivitis are common in patients who are HLA-B27 positive.

Oral Lesions

Oral lesions are recorded in 2.5% of patients and are more common in pustular psoriasis. They manifest as:
- Geographic tongue
- Annular lesions
- Erythematous areas

Dermatopathic Enteropathy

Erythroderma and generalized pustular psoriasis may be associated with enteropathy. This may interfere with systemic absorption of nutrients and drugs.

Death

Death due to psoriasis is uncommon but can occur due to:
- *Erythroderma*: Due to temperature dysregulation, high output cardiac failure and sepsis.
- *Generalized pustular psoriasis*: Due to hypocalcemia which may lead to tetany or cardiac complications.
- *Complications of arthritis*: Arthritis may make patient bed ridden and prone to thrombosis and thromboembolism.
- *Side effects of drugs*: Rarely patient may succumb to side effects of drugs (used for the treatment of severe psoriasis) such as leukopenia, thrombocytopenia, immunosuppression (leading to sepsis), and hepatic and renal damage.

Treatment-related Comorbidities

The management of psoriasis with systemic therapies, while effective, may result in treatment-related comorbidities.
- *Hepatotoxicity*: Notably associated with methotrexate and cyclosporine, necessitating routine liver function assessments.
- *Dyslipidemia*: Observed with the use of cyclosporine and acitretin, indicating the need for lipid profile monitoring.
- *Hypertension*: A potential side effect of cyclosporine use, requiring blood pressure monitoring.
- *Nephrotoxicity*: Particularly relevant to cyclosporine therapy, underscores the importance of renal function evaluation.

Section 2

Diagnosis and Treatment

Investigations

Introduction

Diagnosis of psoriasis is usually clinical, and no investigations need to be done unless:
- Clinical diagnosis is in doubt.
- Patient has complications.
- Patient has to be put on systemic therapy.
- An underlying metabolic syndrome is suspected.

Hematological and Biochemical Parameters

- Usually no change
- *In pustular psoriasis*:
  - Polymorphonuclear leukocytosis as high as 20,000/µL
  - Elevated erythrocyte sedimentation rate (ESR)
  - Hypocalcemia
- *In erythrodermic psoriasis*:
  - Hyperuricemia
  - Hypoproteinemia

Histopathology

Basic Pathological Changes (Figs. 7.1A and B)

Epidermal Changes

- Hyperkeratosis; parakeratosis with focal orthokeratosis
- Thin or absent granular layer with suprapapillary thinning of epidermis
- Regular acanthosis and elongation of rete ridges, which are often clubbed, branched, and frequently fused at their bases.

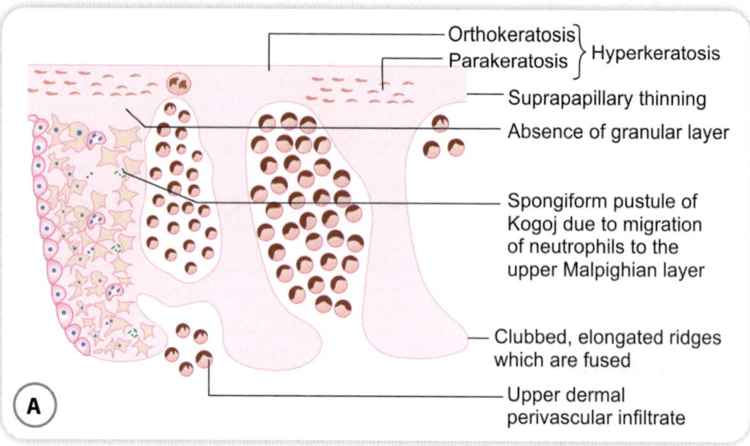

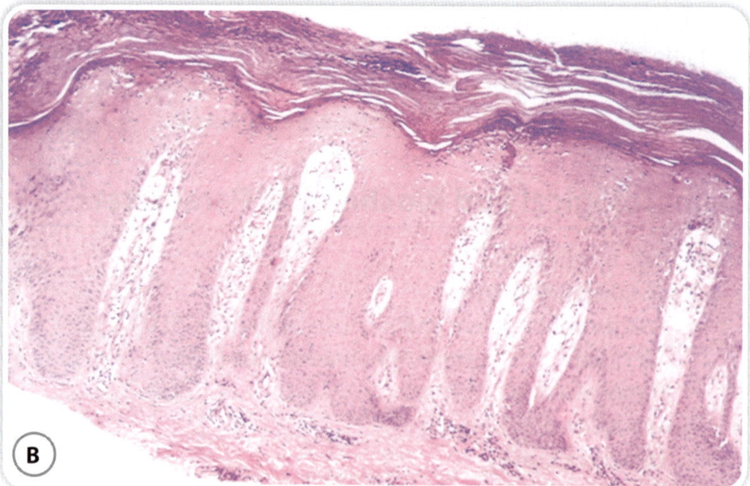

Figs. 7.1A and B: Psoriasis histopathology reveals epidermal hyperkeratosis, parakeratosis, and absent granular layer with thin epidermis above dilated capillary loops. Acanthosis with elongated, often clubbed, rete ridges, and spongiform pustules or Munro's microabscesses due to neutrophil migration are also observed. The dermis displays perivascular infiltrates with mononuclear cells, neutrophils, and extravasated red cells.

- Papillomatosis
- Migration of neutrophils to the upper Malpighian layer (stratum spinosum) to form aggregates within the interstices between the degenerated and thinned keratinocytes (spongiform pustule of Kogoj).

- When these small collections of neutrophils migrate to stratum corneum, they are called *Munro's microabscesses.*

Dermal Changes

- Dilated tortuous papillary dermal capillaries, almost touching stratum corneum, due to suprapapillary thinning
- Perivascular mixed mononuclear and neutrophilic infiltrate admixed with extravasated red cells

Pustular Psoriasis (Figs. 7.2A and B)

Changes seen in pustular psoriasis include:

- Parakeratosis
- Intense papillary and epidermal edema causing spongiosis
- Elongation of rete ridges
- Spongiform pustule of Kogoj.
- Minimal spongiform pustule in the lateral wall of the macro-pustule
- Perivascular mononuclear infiltrate in the upper dermis

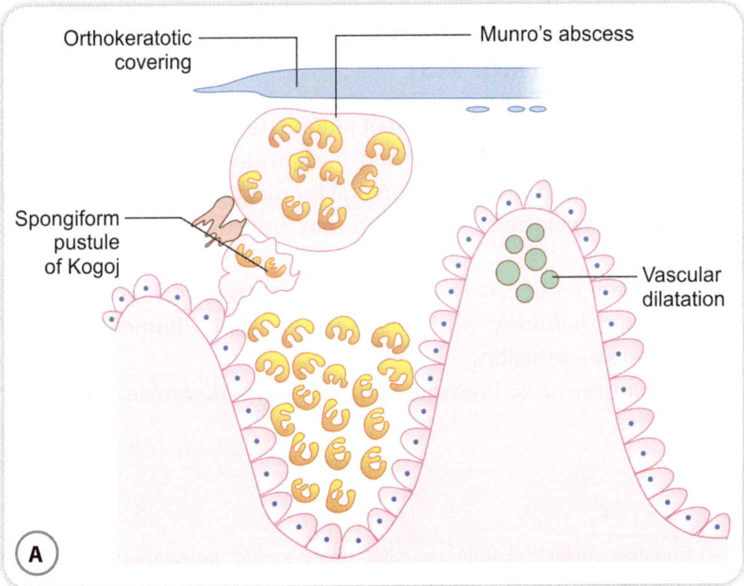

Figs. 7.2A and B: *Continued*

Continued

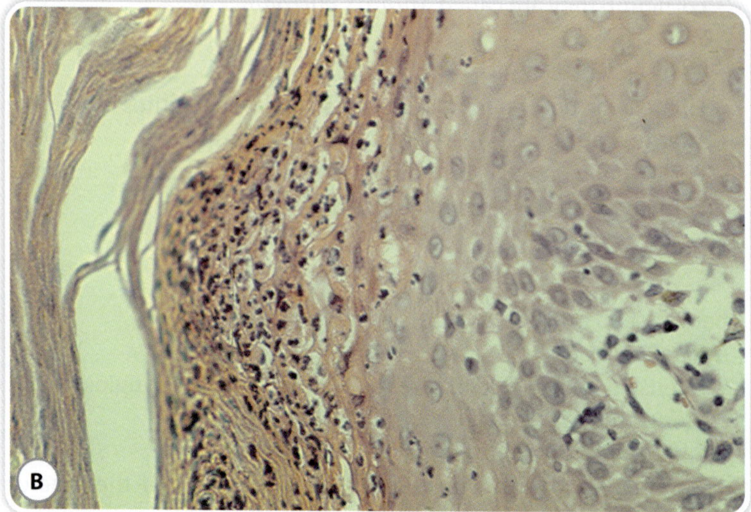

Figs. 7.2A and B: Pustular psoriasis—intense papillary and epidermal edema (spongiosis); spongiform pustule of Kogoj is macroscopic with minimal spongiform pustule in the lateral wall.

Dermoscopy (Fig. 7.3)

The primary dermatoscopic sign of plaque psoriasis includes diffuse white scales over a light, dull red background. Vascular patterns, particularly dotted vessels, are pivotal for diagnosis, becoming more evident after scale removal, which may unveil the dermatoscopic Auspitz sign.[1]

Specific subtypes of psoriasis exhibit variations in scale presence:

- *Psoriatic balanitis and inverse psoriasis*: Characterized by minimal to no scaling.
- *Guttate psoriasis*: Presents with little hyperkeratosis and scant scaling.

---

[1] Dermoscopic Auspitz sign in psoriasis refers to the appearance of pinpoint bleeding spots after scale removal, observed under dermoscopy. It aligns with the histopathologic feature of dilated capillary loops within elongated dermal papillae and is considered a diagnostic clue in psoriasis.

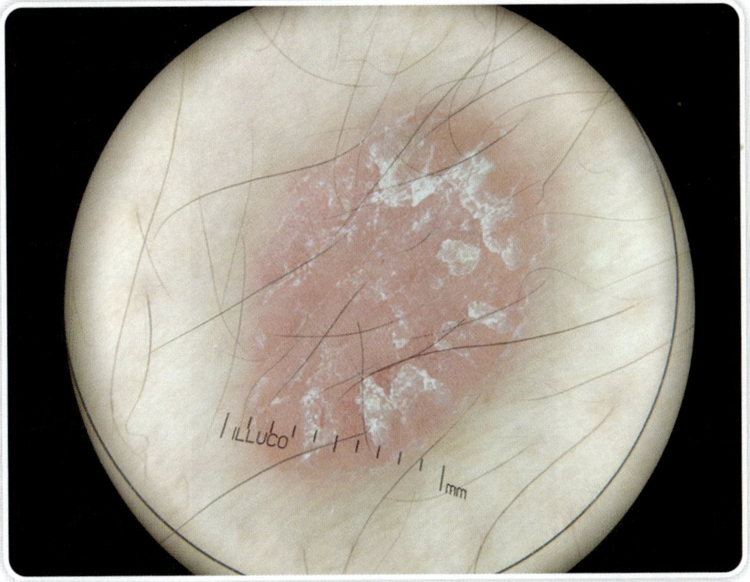

Fig. 7.3: Dermoscopy of psoriasis showing diffuse white scales over erythematous background.

- *Scalp and palmoplantar psoriasis*: Thick hyperkeratotic scales obscure vascular structures, visible post-scale removal.
- *Pustular psoriasis*: Exhibits yellow globules or pustules and crusts.

Radiological Changes

Arthritis is seen in about 10% of patients with psoriasis.

Basic Changes (Fig. 7.4)

The simultaneous presence of ankylosis, periosteal new bone formation, erosions, and osteolysis is strongly suggestive of psoriasis.

Special Changes

In Distal Interphalangeal Type (Fig. 7.5)

Four typical signs seen are:
1. Destructive distal interphalangeal arthropathy with ankylosis
2. Destruction of interphalangeal joints with increased joint space

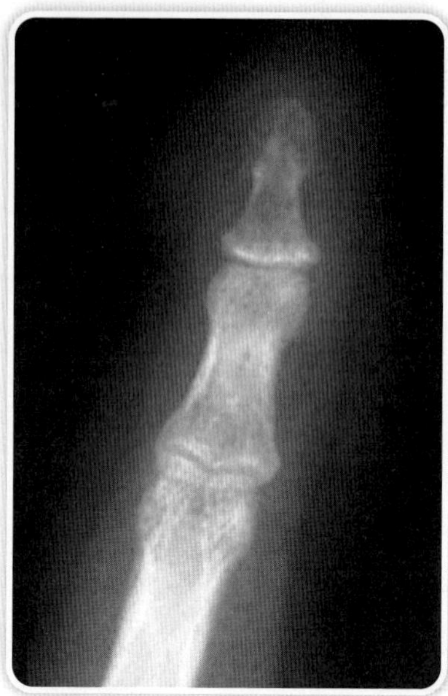

Fig. 7.4: Distal interphalangeal type of psoriatic arthritis—erosions involving distal end of middle phalanx with loss of joint space and associated soft tissue thickening.

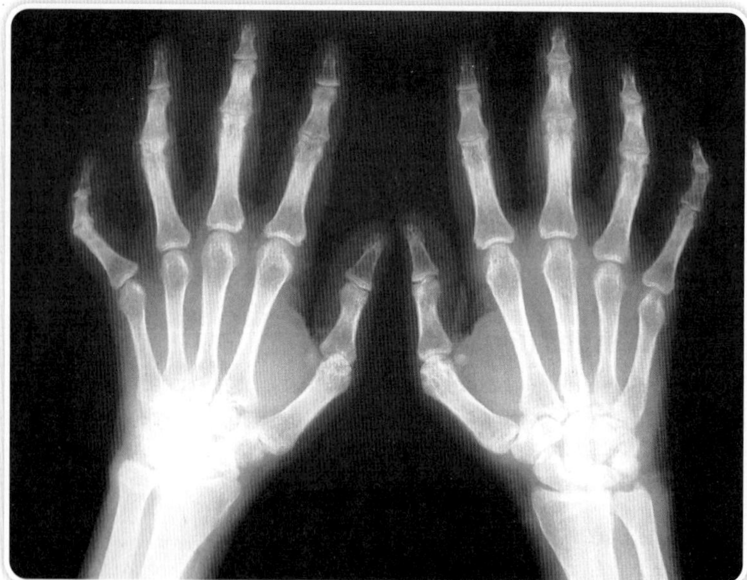

Fig. 7.5: Radiological changes in psoriasis—simultaneous presence of ankylosis, periosteal new bone formation, erosions, and osteolysis is strongly suggestive of psoriasis.

3. Destruction of interphalangeal joint of great toe with bony proliferation of distal phalanx
4. Resorption of tufts of distal phalanx of hand.

In Arthritis Mutilans

- Opera glass hands
- Sharpened pencil appearance due to loss of heads of metatarsal bones

Differential Diagnosis

Introduction

Despite its distinct clinical features, psoriasis can often mimic or be confused with a variety of other dermatological conditions. Accurate diagnosis is crucial for effective management and treatment, necessitating a thorough understanding of the differential diagnoses.

Plaque Psoriasis

Points for Diagnosis

Psoriasis is characterized by:
- Plaques, which are:
  - Well-demarcated, indurated, and erythematous with clear-cut borders.
  - Surmounted with nonadherent, lamellar silvery scales. If scaling is minimal, it can be accentuated by scraping the lesion with a glass slide (*Grattage test*)
  - Scales may be absent in flexures.
  - Positive Auspitz sign.
- Nail changes, characteristic
- Arthritis

Differential Diagnosis

Plaque psoriasis should be differentiated from:

a. Nummular eczema

Nummular eczema (Fig. 8.1)	Psoriasis
Itching extreme	Itching variable
Less well-defined	Well-defined plaques
Papulovesicles, exudative, or lichenified plaques. Induration minimal or nil	Well-defined, erythematous, scaly, indurated plaques
Surmounted with crusts	Surmounted with silvery scales

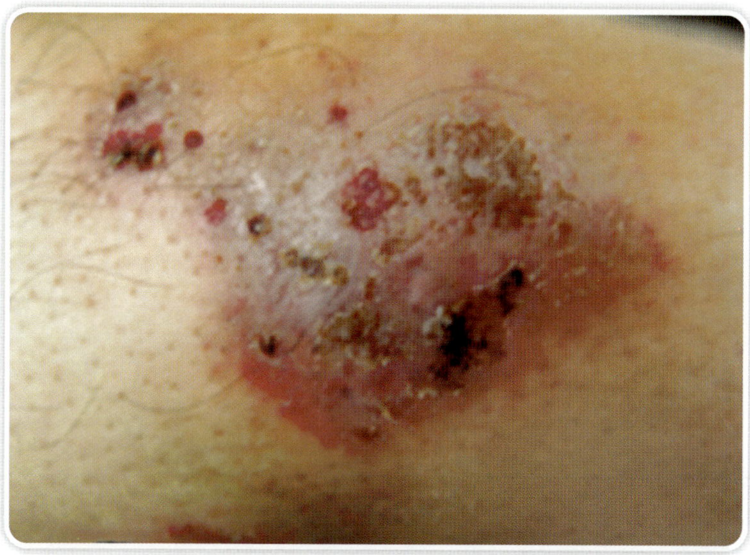

Fig. 8.1: Nummular dermatitis presents less-defined, nonindurated plaques, often lichenified, and exudative, with a characteristic crusting.

b. Pityriasis rubra pilaris (PRP)

PRP (Fig. 8.2)	Psoriasis
Erythematous follicular papules, coalescing to form plaques	Well-defined, erythematous, papules, coalescing to form indurated plaques
Orange-yellow palmoplantar keratoderma, called keratotic sandals	Well-defined, scaly, (usually adherent) erythematous plaques
Nails, discolored, and thickened	Nails show typical changes

c. Mycosis fungoides

Mycosis fungoides (Fig. 8.3)	Psoriasis
Longer history of persistent lesions	Long/short history of lesions characterized by relapses and remissions
Scaling variable	Scaling consistent, except in flexures. Typically, silvery, and removable
Grattage test and Auspitz sign negative	Grattage test and Auspitz sign positive
Lymphadenopathy significant	Absent. Dermatopathic lymphadenopathy seen in erythroderma

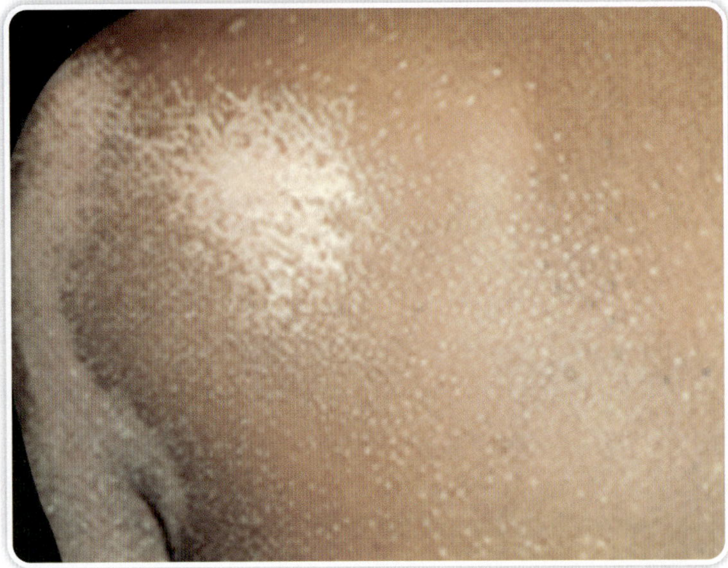

Fig. 8.2: Pityriasis rubra pilaris—erythematous follicular papules, coalescing to form plaques. Often associated with orange-yellow palmoplantar keratoderma, called keratotic sandals.

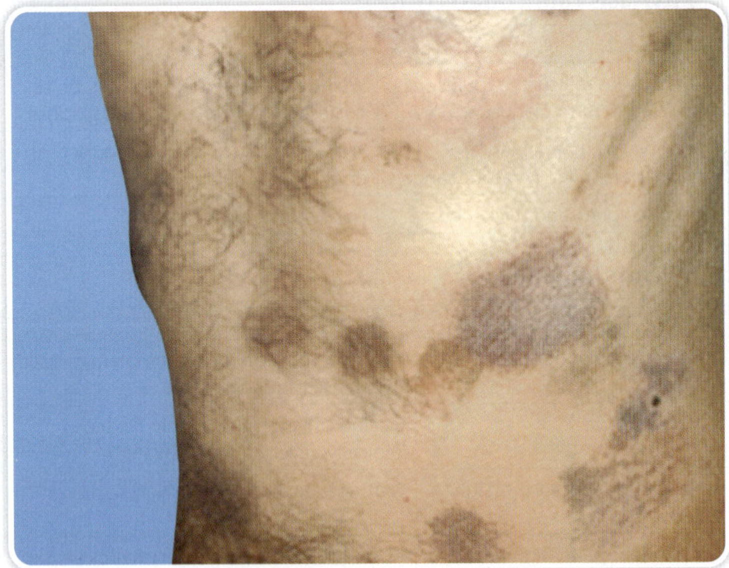

Fig. 8.3: Mycosis fungoides: Persistent indurated lesions with variable scaling. Grattage test and Auspitz sign negative. There may be significant lymphadenopathy.

d. Seborrheic dermatitis of scalp

Seborrheic dermatitis of scalp (Fig. 8.4)	Scalp psoriasis
Itching severe	Itching variable
Less well-defined plaques. Minimal or no induration	Well-defined, erythematous, indurated plaques
Greasy scales	Silvery scales, often heaped up
No spillage on forehead and nape of neck	Spillage on forehead and nape of neck

e. Flexural seborrheic dermatitis

Flexural seborrheic dermatitis (Fig. 8.5)	Flexural psoriasis
Itching severe	Itching variable
Less well-defined, scaly/crusted plaques. Minimal or no induration	Well-defined, indurated plaques

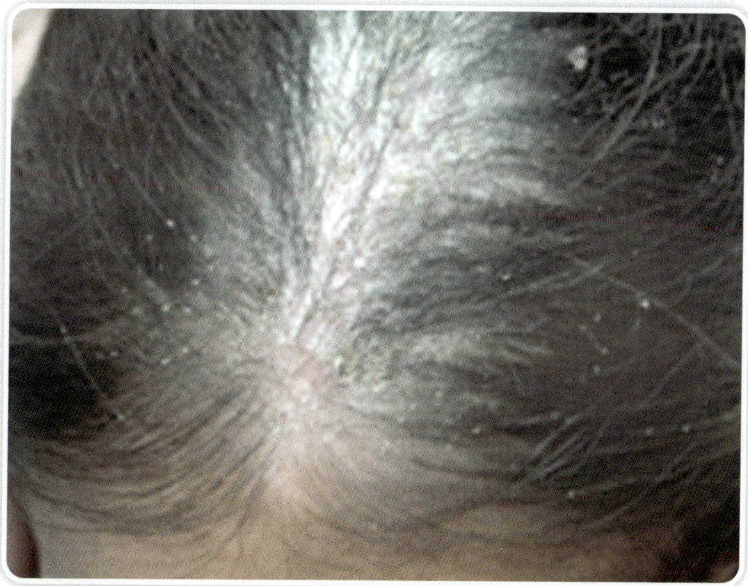

Fig. 8.4: Seborrheic dermatitis of scalp—less well-defined plaques with minimal or no induration. Surmounted by greasy scales. Note that there is no spillage on the forehead and nape of neck.

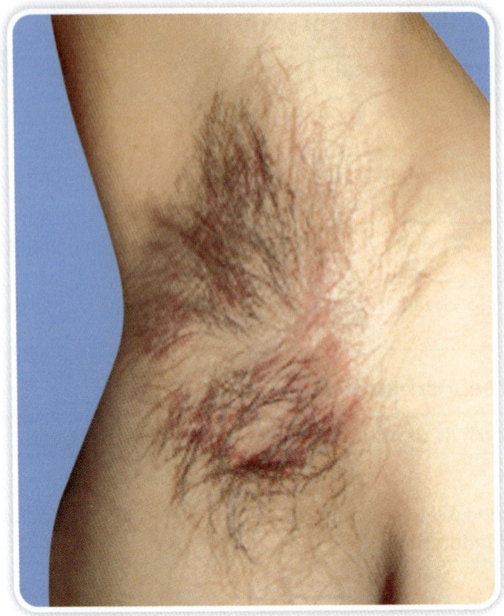

Fig. 8.5: Seborrheic dermatitis in flexures—less well-defined scaly/crusted plaques with minimal or no induration and erythema.

f. Hyperkeratotic hand eczema

Hyperkeratotic hand eczema (Fig. 8.6)	Palmoplantar psoriasis
Itching severe	Itching variable
Less well-defined plaques. Minimal or no induration	Well-defined, erythematous, indurated plaques
Plaques surmounted with vesicles, crusts, and yellow scales	Plaques surmounted with silvery scales
No spillage on to the wrist	Often extends proximal to the wrist
Knuckles not involved	Knuckles often thickened

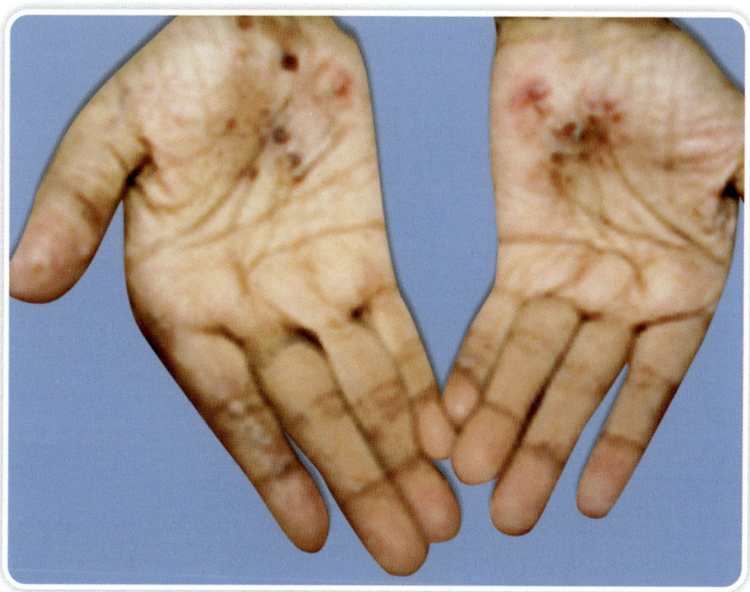

Fig. 8.6: Hyperkeratotic hand eczema—less well-defined plaques with minimal or no induration. Plaques surmounted with vesicles, crusts, and yellow scales and there is no spillage onto the wrist.

Guttate Psoriasis

Points for Diagnosis

Guttate psoriasis is characterized by:
- Papules which are small (drop-like), discrete, and scattered.
- Salmon-pink and surmounted with scales. Scales, if absent, can be accentuated by scraping the lesion with a glass slide.
- Lesions present predominantly on trunk.

Differential Diagnosis

Guttate psoriasis should be differentiated from:

a. **Pityriasis lichenoides chronica (PLC)**

PLC (Fig. 8.7)	Guttate psoriasis
Erythematous papules which are small and discrete	Salmon-pink papules which are small (drop-like), discrete, and scattered
Micaceous scales, which can be removed in toto	Lamellar non-adherent scales. Scales, if absent, can be accentuated by scraping lesion with glass slide
Subside with hypopigmentation	Subside with hypo/hyperpigmentation

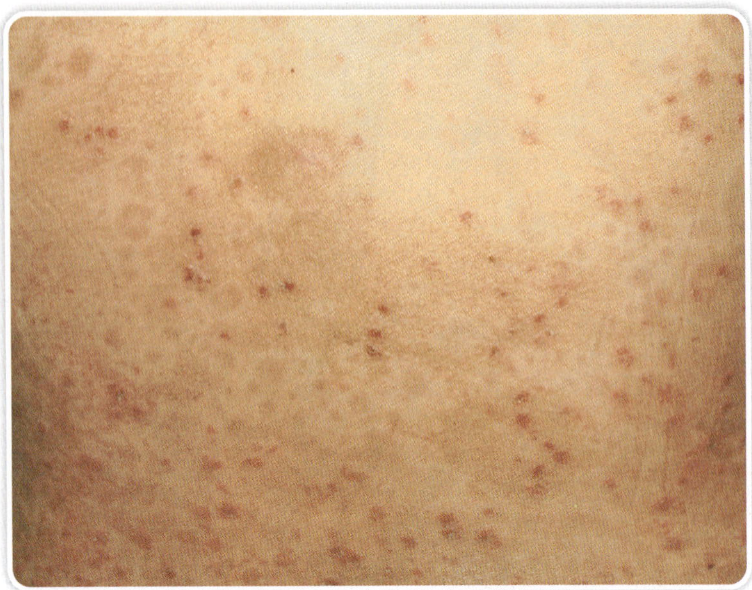

Fig. 8.7: Pityriasis lichenoides chronica—erythematous small and discrete papules surmounted with mica like scales, which can be removed in toto. Lesions subside with hypopigmentation.

b. Secondary syphilis

Secondary syphilis (Fig. 8.8)	Guttate psoriasis
Morphology variable—one type papulosquamous	Salmon-pink papules which are small (drop-like), discrete, and scattered
Variable scaling. Auspitz sign negative	Lamellar, nonadherent scales. Scales, if absent, can be accentuated by scraping the lesion with a glass slide. Auspitz sign positive
Lesions predominantly truncal, facial, and present on palms and soles	Lesions truncal. Face, palms and soles spared
Mucosal lesions, lymphadenopathy, and perianal lesions frequent	Not seen

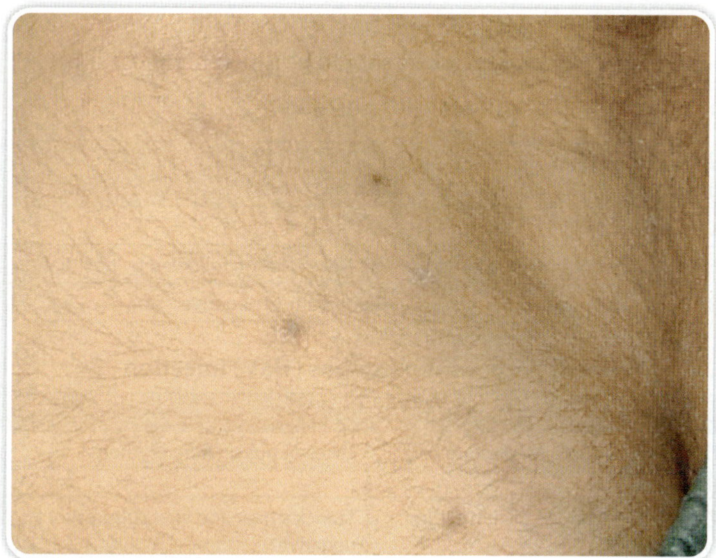

Fig. 8.8: Secondary syphilis—one type, papulosquamous. Papules with variable scaling. Auspitz sign negative. Lesions predominantly on trunk, face, and present on palms and soles. Mucosal lesions, lymphadenopathy, and perianal lesions frequent.

Generalized Pustular Psoriasis

Points for Diagnosis

Generalized pustular psoriasis (GPP) is characterized by:
- Sudden appearance of fiery red erythema, initially patchy, soon becoming confluent and generalized. Within a few hours, a cluster of tiny, nonfollicular, very superficial creamy-white pustules develop. The pustules either become confluent, forming circinate lesions, and "lakes of pus" or are literally wiped off (because they are superficial) resulting in red-oozing erosions.
- Lesions crust and as the crusts are shed, new crops of pustules may appear at the same site. Characteristically, new pustules appear in waves, usually accompanied by fever.
- Nikolsky's sign may be positive in the untreated patient.[1]

---

[1] Nikolsky's sign is traditionally associated with blistering skin conditions such as pemphigus vulgaris. In the context of generalized pustular psoriasis (GPP), a positive Nikolsky's sign indicates the ease with which the top layers of the skin can be dislodged, due to the fragile nature of the skin overlying pustules and erythematous areas. This sign helps differentiate GPP from other pustular diseases and indicates the severity of epidermal involvement.

Differential Diagnosis

Generalized pustular psoriasis should be differentiated from:

a. Widespread erythema with pustules

Widespread erythema with pustules	GPP
Less acute	Acute
Evolution not typical erythema	Typical evolution followed by pustulation
Blood culture positive	Blood culture negative

b. Generalized herpes simplex virus (HSV) infection

Generalized HSV infection (Fig. 8.9)	GPP
Umbilicated pustules, discrete and grouped	Lakes of pus on fiery erythema
Tzanck smear and viral cultures for HSV positive	Tzanck smear and viral cultures for HSV negative

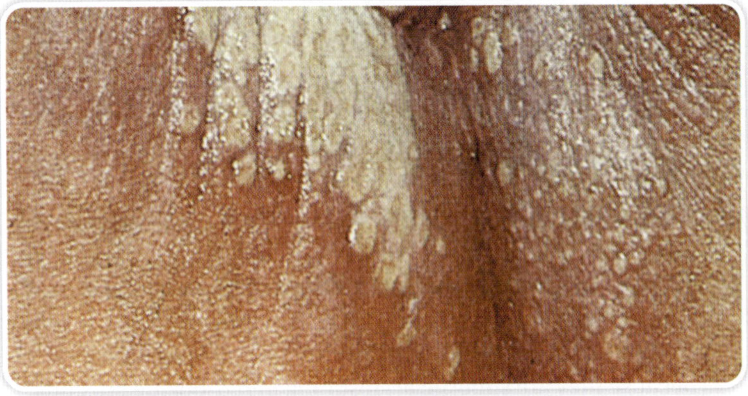

Fig. 8.9: Generalized herpes simplex—umbilicated pustules, discrete and grouped.

c. Acute generalized pustular drug eruption

Acute generalized pustular drug eruption	GPP
Occurs after intake of furosemide, amoxicillin/clavulanic acid, etc.	May occur after withdrawal of corticosteroids
Clinically similar, but patients are less toxic	Patients are very toxic

Nail Psoriasis

Points for Diagnosis

Nail psoriasis is characterized by:
- Pitting of the nail plate
- Oil spot sign
- Onycholysis
- Subungual hyperkeratosis
- Discoloration of nail plate
- Onychodystrophy
- Anonychia

Differential Diagnosis

Nail psoriasis should be differentiated from:

Onychomycosis:

Onychomycosis (Fig. 8.10)	Nail psoriasis
Thickened nail plate typically shows tunneling and friable subungual debris	Thickened nail plate does not show tunneling
Pitting uncommon	Pitting common
Potassium hydroxide mount positive for fungus	Potassium hydroxide mount negative for fungus, unless a secondary invader

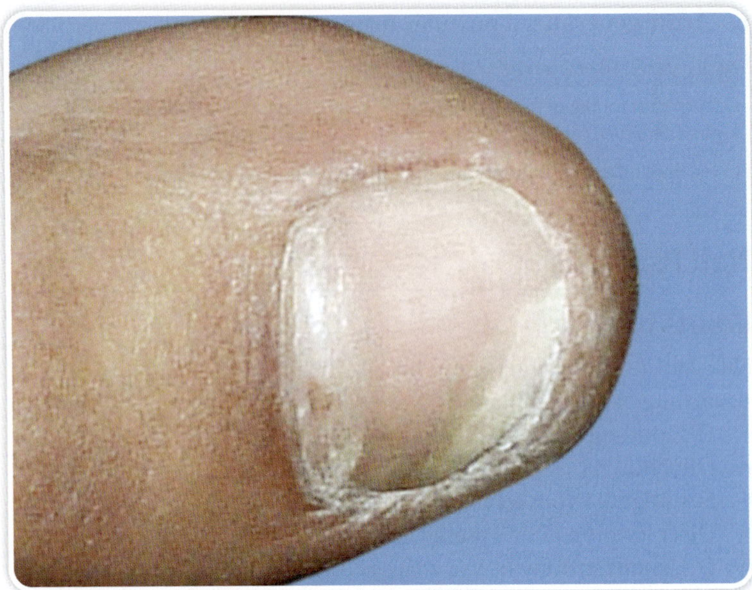

Fig. 8.10: Onychomycosis—thickened nail plate typically shows tunneling and subungual debris which is friable. Pitting is not present. Potassium hydroxide mount is positive for fungus.

General Principles of Treatment

Introduction

The treatment of psoriasis seeks to attain long-term disease management, alleviate symptoms, enhance quality of life, and mitigate the risk of associated comorbidities. This necessitates a holistic approach encompassing patient education, lifestyle changes, topical treatments, phototherapy, systemic therapies, and biologic agents.

Factors which Determine Treatment

Treatment of every patient should be individualized and depends on several factors:

- *Patient factors*:
  - Age of patient
  - Gender
  - Occupation of patient
  - Psyche of patient
  - Resources available
- *Disease factors*:
  - Duration of disease
  - *Extent*: Percentage of body surface area involved and whether important sites such as palms, soles, scalp, and face are affected.
  - *Type of psoriasis*: Whether chronic plaque/guttate/erythroderma/generalized pustular/palmoplantar psoriasis, etc.
  - Natural history of disease in the patient
  - Nail changes and joint involvement
- *Social factors*:
  - Effect of disease on the patient's quality of life
  - Acceptance of disease by the family/society

Information to Patient (See Annexure 4)

The following information should be made available to all patients:
- Information on available treatment options, including expense of treatment. Hospital- or clinic-based treatments should be planned in a way that minimizes disruption to the patient's routine.
- Realistic treatment outcomes/expectations should be discussed. It should be clarified to the patient that the aim of treatment is to control the disease, so that normal physical and social function is resumed. It may be prudent to tell the patient that all treatment options available can induce remissions and do not prevent relapses.

Instructions to Patients

Patients should be advised about:
- Alcohol and smoking restrictions
- No dietary restrictions[1]

Treatment Options

Treatment options available in psoriasis include:
- Topical therapy (Chapter 10)
- Phototherapy and photochemotherapy (Chapter 11).
- Systemic therapy (Chapter 12)
- Biologicals therapy (Chapter 13)
- The medications may be prescribed in combination, rotation, or sequentially (Chapter 14).

---

[1] While no specific dietary restrictions are necessary for the treatment of psoriasis itself, patients with metabolic syndrome or those attempting weight loss should aim for a diet low in saturated fats and sugars.

Topical Therapy

Introduction

Topical therapy is the mainstay of therapy in localized psoriasis [body surface area (BSA) <10%] and in patients with extensive disease associated with comorbidities, which preclude the use of systemic therapy. It is also used as adjunctive therapy in patients with extensive disease (BSA >10%).

Several topical agents are available:
- Emollients
- Coal tar (CT)
- Dithranol
- Calcipotriol
- Corticosteroids
- Retinoids
- Methotrexate
- Newer agents

  In psoriasis, the topical agents may be used as monotherapy (less frequently) or in combination with other topical/systemic agents.

Emollients

Emollients are the main adjuvant therapy used in patients with psoriasis of all severities.

Mode of Action

- Emollients reduce scaling and itching, both bothersome symptoms in patients with psoriasis.
- They restore stratum corneum barrier function.

- They are also applied to lesions of psoriasis before exposure to ultraviolet rays (UVR) to produce a uniform interface between scales and reduce scattering of light.

Use in Psoriasis

Emollients are indicated as:
- *Monotherapy*:
  - To treat limited number of lesions
  - To manage mild relapses
- *As adjuncts*:
  - In all patients, especially those in erythroderma
  - In patients on phototherapy and photochemotherapy, prior to exposure to UVR to reduce scattering of light

Preparations Available

Petrolatum[1]

- *Advantages*:
  - Good emollient with long (several hours) period of effect
  - Easily available over-the-counter
  - Inexpensive
  - Patient can be educated to manage limited/mild relapses on his/her own.
  - Staining of clothes is mild and the stains are usually washable.
- *Disadvantages*:
  - Messy to use
  - Feels sticky, particularly in summers
  - Irritation, if of poor quality
  - Chemical folliculitis or pustular lesions due to occlusive effect

Coconut Oil

- In India, coconut oil is commonly used as an emollient in psoriasis.
- It has mild emollient effect, which lasts only for a few hours.

---

[1] *Petrolatum*: Product of fractional distillation of petroleum. One market brand—Vaseline.

Cold Cream

Cold cream is as effective as petrolatum, but duration of effect is shorter.

- *Advantages*:
  - Cosmetically better tolerated
  - Creams containing urea have added advantage, as urea is both a hygroscopic and a keratolytic agent.
- *Disadvantages*:
  - Expensive
  - Shorter duration of effect than petrolatum
  - It may contain unnecessary ingredients such as perfumes, herbs, and lightening agents, which not only add to the cost but may have undesirable effects. Fragrances can cause sensitivity. Extract of aloe vera, which is gaining popularity and is present in several creams, probably has little effect on psoriasis, though it adds to cost.

Application

- Frequency of application of emollients depends on the degree of scaling. Generally 2–3 applications a day are sufficient.
- If there are few lesions, then emollients are applied only on lesions, but if the lesions are multiple, then the applications are made on the entire area rather than only on the lesional skin for convenience of application.
- Best applied after a soaking bath. Or after soaking part affected (as in palms and soles). Or after application of soaks.

Tars

Tars are one of the most widely used topical agents in the treatment of psoriasis.

Properties

Tars are produced by destructive distillation[2] of substances like wood, shale, and coal. Among the various types of tars, CT is the most widely used in psoriasis.

---

[2] *Destructive distillation*: Heating a substance in the absence of air.

Coal Tar

- CT is prepared by destructive distillation of bituminous coal.[3]
- CT is a mixture of thousands of hydrocarbons with different aromatic components, such as benzols, naphthalene, and anthracenes.

Shale Tar

- Shale tar is prepared by destructive distillation of shale[4] deposits (in the sea), e.g., ichthammol or ichthyol.
- It is a black viscous liquid containing ammonium salts of sulfonic acids and ammonium sulfate.

Mode of Action

Coal tar is an essential component of several treatment protocols for psoriasis, but its mode of action has not been elucidated.

- Though CT by itself is effective in psoriasis, conventionally it has been used in combination with ultraviolet light. CT sensitizes skin to ultraviolet A (UVA) and not to UVB, but interestingly, it is a combination of UVB with CT which is more effective, in treatment of psoriasis.
- CT has a cytostatic effect and combination of CT with UVR reduces epidermal DNA synthesis in psoriasis.

Use in Psoriasis

Indications

Coal tar is indicated in:

- Plaque psoriasis, involving < 20% BSA
- Guttate psoriasis evolving into plaque psoriasis
- Few lesions persisting after systemic therapy

Contraindications

Coal tar preparations are best avoided in:

- Flexures
- Unstable psoriasis, pustular psoriasis, and erythrodermic psoriasis

---

[3] *Bituminous coal*: Coal is of four types—Anthracite, bituminous, lignite, and peat.
[4] *Shale*: It is a type of rock.

Treatment Protocols

Goeckerman Regimen

- *Historical background*: Goeckerman in 1925 at Mayo clinic developed a protocol for treating psoriasis using application of crude CT followed by exposure to UVR. The original Goeckerman regimen has been modified and is now practiced in its modified form, at several centers.
- *Method*: It consists of application of CT followed by exposure to UV light. The regimen is practiced either in hospitalized patients or in day-care centers, as it requires supervision and needs assistance of a nursing staff:
  - Used either as 3% crude CT in petrolatum. Or as 5% refined tar with 3% ichthyol and 10% Tween 80 in petrolatum.
  - Applied three times a day, on entire body surface except in flexures where either 1% hydrocortisone cream or a mild water-soluble emollient is used. Scalp is treated with 10–20% liquor picis carbonis in oil.
  - After 24-hours, excess tar is removed using vegetable oil such as corn or cotton seed oil and entire skin is exposed to 70% of minimal erythema dose (MED)[5] of UVB using UVB lamps.
  - *For UVB exposure, body is divided into eight zones*: Two on posterior, two on anterior, and two each on lateral surface. Scalp, if involved, is exposed separately. On thick plaques, additional exposure is given.
  - After UVB exposure, the body is cleansed using lukewarm water and soap to remove tar, scales, epithelial debris, and bacteria while the scalp is washed with shampoo.
  - An hour later, tar is reapplied for the next day. Depending on the erythema response, dose of UVB is either omitted (if the erythema is marked), continued at previous dose (if the erythema is marginal) or increased by 20% (if the erythema is minimal).
  - Total 3–5 treatments a week are given.

---

[5] *MED*: Minimum dose of UVB required to produce just perceptible erythema. The erythema should develop within 4–6 hours and disappear by 24 hours.

- *Response*:
  - It is seen within 2–3 weeks.
  - Leads to remission in 80% of patients after approximately 30 treatments.
  - Remission maintained by intermittent therapy given 1–2 times a week.

Modified Goeckerman Regimen

Basic protocol has been modified for the convenience of patients:

- Application of ointment containing CT with or without salicylic acid, at home by the patients themselves, is the most widely used treatment modality for psoriasis. Salicylic acid (3%) is added to CT to improve its penetration and for its keratolytic action. On palms and soles, a higher concentration (up to 6%) may be used.
- Ultraviolet ray exposure may be given on an outpatient basis, 1–2 hours after application of CT in petrolatum or alternatively the patient may be advised to expose to sunlight.

Advantages

- Coal tar does not cause allergic contact dermatitis.
- It also does not have any carcinogenic properties,[6] though this had been a major concern earlier.

Disadvantages

- Coal tar in petrolatum base is black in color and is messy to use, because it stains clothes and has an unpleasant odor (though mild). Recently, some colorless products containing CT have been produced. Though cosmetically better accepted, their clinical efficacy needs to be evaluated. It is believed that the more cruder and darker the CT, the more efficacious it is.
- Since CT is a mixture, it is difficult to standardize the concentration of its ingredients and hence the response to treatment of psoriasis with two different batches of CT is likely to be different.
- Some CTs may cause irritation.

---

[6] *Carcinogenic potential*: The small increased risk of malignancies in patients receiving Goeckerman regimen is related to the concomitant exposure to UVB.

Preparations Available

Coal tar is available in various concentrations, formulations, and combinations for treatment of psoriasis:

- *CT tar ointment*:[7] It contains 6% CT with 3% salicylic acid in petrolatum and is the most widely used preparation.
- *CT paste*:[8] It contains 7.5% CT in compound zinc paste.
- *CT solution (liquor picis carbonis)*:[9] It is prepared by extracting CT in the presence of polysorbate 80 with alcohol. CT solution is less messy than original CT but is also less efficacious. CT solution has the advantage of having a mild antipruritic action.
- *CT shampoo*: It is available for use on hairy areas, such as scalp. However, such preparations, unless left on the scalp for a reasonable period (preferably overnight), only have a cleansing effect. Therefore, CT solution (without shampoo) is preferred as an overnight application followed by shampooing, the next morning.
- *Exorex®*: A new topical lotion, containing CT 1%, is reported to be as effective as CT ointment, when used 2–3 times/day.

Dithranol (Anthranil)

History

- Squire (1877), first described the beneficial effect of extract of *Andira araroba* in psoriasis.
- Unna (1916) first used dithranol
- Ingram standardized anthralin regimen in psoriasis

Properties

Chrysarobin is the active principle in the extract of *A. araroba* and dithranol is its synthetic derivative, in which the methyl group located at C3 in chrysarobin is replaced by hydrogen. Dithranol is yellow-orange in color.

---

[7] *Ointment*: A grease of soft consistency used as a base to which CT has been added.
[8] *Paste*: Stiffer, less greasy and less occlusive than ointment.
[9] *Solution*: Dissolution of one or more substances into homogeneous clarity in a liquid vehicle (which can be aqueous, alcoholic, or hydroalcoholic).

Mode of Action

Dithranol acts in psoriasis because it:

- Has a strong anti-inflammatory action.
- Reduces keratinocyte proliferation by releasing free radicals impeding DNA replication.

Indications

Dithranol is indicated in the following situations:

- Chronic plaque psoriasis, with a few large plaques
- Palmoplantar psoriasis
- Resistant scalp psoriasis but can discolor blonde hair

Treatment Protocols

The use of dithranol requires detailed instructions to the patient on careful application of medication. Several regimens are available.

Short Contact Therapy

- Dithranol 1–5% is used, beginning with 1%.
- Dithranol ointment is carefully applied to the psoriatic lesions, using an applicator. Application to the surrounding normal skin is avoided by applying petrolatum.
- After 10–30 minutes, excess ointment is removed with a clean applicator and washed off with soap and water. Washing with 1% KOH or triethanolamine cream produces better removal of dithranol, reducing irritation.
- If no erythema develops on surrounding skin:
  - Daily application is continued at same concentration and application time is increased weekly.
  - Or the concentration is increased weekly and contact time kept constant.
- If erythema develops, a lower concentration of dithranol is used and the application time is increased weekly.

Ingram Regimen

This protocol is rarely used in India.

- Dithranol (in lower concentration of 0.05–0.1%) is applied as Lassar's paste,[10] at night.

---

[10] *Lassar's paste*: It contains dithranol and salicylic acid in zinc paste.

- Excess paste and scales are removed in morning with oil followed by a tar bath for 20 minutes and UVB irradiation, using UVB lamps.
- It is followed by reapplication of dithranol.

Combination Regimens

- *With corticosteroids*: Use of a corticosteroid cream (fluocinonide, 0.05% or betamethasone valerate, 0.1%) during the day and dithranol at night reduces the irritation, brings about rapid relief but does not increase period of remission.
- *With calcipotriol or UVB*: Dithranol can be combined with calcipotriol or UVB and the combination is more effective than dithranol alone.

Advantages

- Absence of any long-term side effects allows for unlimited use of drug, whenever lesions recur.
- No increased risk of skin cancers.

Side Effects

Irritant Dermatitis

Dithranol causes irritant dermatitis either in susceptible individuals or if the concentration is increased rapidly.

Patient complains of burning sensation and develops erythema, which peaks at 3 days after single application. Rarely, bullae may develop.

Redness of distant sites, like face, may develop because of accidental transfer of the drug from hands. So, it is essential to wash hands after application.

Discoloration

Brown discoloration of surrounding skin[11] is frequent and is due to products of oxidation. Washing with 1% KOH or triethanolamine cream produces better removal of dithranol, reducing pigmentation.

---

[11] *Discoloration*: Discoloration of hands can be avoided by using gloves and avoiding hot water to wash and instead using cold or luke warm water.

Once pigmentation develops, it fades over a period of time, because the oxidation products are deposited only in stratum corneum.

Dithranol also causes discoloration (purple or green) of hair, so it should not be used as first-line therapy for scalp psoriasis.

Dithranol also stains clothes and these are difficult to remove.

Preparations

Dithranol is available as:

- *Derobin ointment containing*:
  - Dithranol, 1.15%
  - Coal tar[12] solution, 5.3%
  - Salicylic acid,[13] 1.15%
  - Petrolatum base
- *Micanol* (0.1, 1%) a new cream-based preparation, has comparative efficacy and stains clothes much less.
- New formulations in emulsifying ointment base with 0.1% w/w ascorbyl palmitate as an antioxidant are stable for up to 52 weeks.

Calcipotriol

Properties

- Vitamin D3 (cholecalciferol) is synthesized naturally by epidermal keratinocytes and is metabolized to the biologically active form, 1,25 dihydroxy D3 by the kidneys.
- Though 1,25 dihydroxy D3 has an antipsoriatic effect, its therapeutic effect is limited by its hypercalcemic action.
- Synthetic vitamin D3 analogs have been developed (by modification of the side chain) to enhance the antipsoriatic effect of vitamin D3 and reduce their hypercalcemic action (because they are rapidly transformed into inactive metabolites).
- Calcipotriol (or calcipotriene, as it is called in Europe) and tacalcitol (1,24 dihydroxy vitamin D3) are currently the most promising synthetic analogs.

---

[12] *Coal tar*: It is added to reduce irritation and salicylic acid to stabilize the preparation.
[13] *Salicylic acid*: To stabilize the preparation.

Mode of Action

Calcipotriol attaches to vitamin D receptor (VDR) and this ligand-receptor complex binds to DNA sequences within the vitamin D-responsive genes and exerts antipsoriatic effect by:

- Inhibiting cellular proliferation
- Inducing terminal cell differentiation
- *Exerting anti-inflammatory effects by*:
  - Acting on monocytes, macrophages, B and T-lymphocytes that express the VDR.
  - Reducing dermal cellular infiltrate with a shift from predominantly CD4+ helper cells to CD8+ suppressor cells.
  - Reducing the number of infiltrating neutrophils.

Indications

Calcipotriol is indicated in the following situations:

- *In mild to moderate chronic plaque psoriasis*: Calcipotriol is very effective both as a monotherapy or as combination therapy with dithranol and corticosteroids.
- *In widespread psoriasis*: Calcipotriol is used as an adjuvant with other systemic agents like psoralen plus UVA (PUVA), UVB, or cyclosporine, since combination of systemic therapy with calcipotriol has been found to be more efficacious than systemic therapy alone.

Contraindications

Calcipotriol should be avoided in:

- Unstable, erythrodermic, or pustular psoriasis since its irritating potential may exacerbate the disease.
- In patients with concomitant atopic dermatitis, neurodermatitis, or nummular eczema

Treatment Protocols

Monotherapy

- Calcipotriol ointment (50 mg/g) is applied twice daily on the psoriatic plaques.
- Total weekly dose should not exceed 100 g in adults and 50 g in children.

Combined Topical Therapy

- *With dithranol*:
  - Calcipotriol ointment is applied twice daily and dithranol cream is applied once daily for 30 minutes.
  - Combination is more efficacious than dithranol used alone.
- *With topical corticosteroids*:
  - Used at separate times or as combination therapy. Or using it on weekdays and topical steroids on weekends.
  - Efficacy of both is enhanced and skin irritation due to calcipotriol is reduced.

Combination with Systemic Therapy

- In widespread psoriasis, calcipotriol is used as an adjuvant with other systemic agents like, PUVA, narrow-band UVB (NBUVB), cyclosporine, or acitretin.
- *Combination therapy:* With calcipotriol has been found to be more efficacious than systemic therapy alone.
- When used with phototherapy, calcipotriol should be applied after exposure to UV light. Or it should be applied at least 2 hours before phototherapy because of inactivation of calcipotriol molecule by light.

Precautions

- Calcipotriol should not be used on the face. To avoid accidental contact with the eyes, hands should be washed thoroughly after application.
- Maximum limit of 100 g/week in adults and 50 g/week in children should not be exceeded.
- It should not be mixed with other drugs or vehicles to avoid alteration of pH, as calcipotriol requires a high pH to be stable.
- It is inactivated by salicylic acid, so psoriasis plaques should not be pretreated with salicylic acid.

Response

- Significant improvement is perceptible at the end of first week and marked improvement is observed in majority of patients by 6 weeks.

- Though the drug decreases thickness of plaques, some residual thickness often persists. In such a case, either the ointment is applied under occlusion or supplemented with other topical or systemic agents.

Advantages

- Calcipotriol is well tolerated in pediatric age group.
- It does not induce skin atrophy (*c.f.,* topical corticosteroids).
- It does not photosensitize even on prolonged use.
- It is not teratogenic. If a patient conceives during calcipotriol therapy, the drug should be stopped. However, elective abortion is not indicated. (Pregnancy category C)

Side Effects

Skin Irritation

- Skin irritation occurs approximately in 15% of patients, but only 1–2% of patients need to discontinue treatment.
- It varies from transient burning or stinging sensation (more frequent) to erythema and scaling (less frequent).
- Face is particularly sensitive; facial irritation can occur either due to direct local application or due to transfer of the ointment, applied elsewhere.
- Contact allergic dermatitis to calcipotriol is extremely rare.

Hypercalcemia

- Hypercalcemia is rarely observed with topical therapy and occurs after excessive (weekly dose exceeding 100 g) or prolonged application of calcipotriol, usually in patients with concomitant renal impairment.
- Serum calcium levels normalize within 1 week of stopping therapy.

Preparations

- Calcipotriol (Daivonex® and Psorcutan®) is available as 50 µg/g ointment, cream, and solution internationally, but only as an ointment and solution in India.

- A combination of calcipotriol and betamethasone is also now available in India, in an ointment base (Daivobet®).

Corticosteroids

Corticosteroids should be used in the treatment of the psoriasis with a word of caution, because they are like a double-edged weapon. Though both topical and systemic steroids are effective in psoriasis, their usefulness is often overshadowed by their side effects.

Mode of Action

Corticosteroids have:
- Anti-inflammatory action
- *Antiproliferative action*: Corticosteroids inhibit the progression of epidermal cells from G1 to S phase.
- They decrease the mitotic index, both in psoriasis and normal epidermis. The biological actions of glucocorticosteroids occur at the molecular level (gene transcription and modulation of protein synthesis and nucleic acid metabolism).
- Immunosuppressive action

Indications

The use of topical corticosteroids[14] as monotherapy in treatment of psoriasis should be discouraged, and they are best considered as agents which rapidly reduce the inflammation of psoriasis, while the specific modalities (which have a more gradual onset of action) control disease activity, with fewer side effects. They are easy to use, provide rapid response, and improve the quality of the life.

Topical corticosteroids are frequently used in the treatment of psoriasis for achieving rapid symptomatic relief in:
- *Psoriasis on scalp, face, neck, flexures, and genitals*: Corticosteroids are often used as first line of treatment. On scalp, lotions are preferred and may be combined with tar preparations.
- *Palmoplantar psoriasis*: Corticosteroids are frequently used, combined with salicylic acid and tar in an ointment base.

---

[14] Except in special situations, use of systemic steroids in management of psoriasis is best avoided.

- *Combination therapy*: Calcipotriol ointment as daily application or pulse applications at weekends along with daily application of corticosteroids is aimed at reducing the side effects of each agent and targeted at psoriasis patients who are not accepting tar preparations.

Treatment Protocols

Corticosteroids can be used:
- Undiluted
- Diluted with creams in ratios of 1:1 or 1:2,[15] to make their use cost-effective (for larger areas) and to reduce side effects (on prolonged use).
- Combined with other topical preparations such as salicylic acid, urea, lactic acid, and tar.
- Though the use of topical corticosteroids under occlusion is a convenient and clinically effective way to clear (temporarily) plaque psoriasis, it is not recommended, as the side effects are amplified.
- Intralesional injections of corticosteroids, e.g., triamcinolone acetonide, are a useful technique used to treat troublesome, small, recalcitrant plaques of psoriasis. The effect is long lasting and repetition of the injection is usually unnecessary for several months.

Side Effects

Repeated application of corticosteroids results in a cumulative depot effect in the skin and increased side effects as well as increased systemic absorption.

Newer topical corticosteroids preparations such as fluticasone propionate, mometasone furoate, and prednicarbate have fewer side effects.

Long-term use of topical steroids can be associated with the following side effects:
- *Tachyphylaxis*: It has also been observed that continuous use of topical corticosteroids leads to diminished therapeutic response due to tachyphylaxis.

---

[15] *1:2*: It means 1 part of steroid and 2 parts of cold cream.

- *Cutaneous changes*: Prolonged use of topical steroids results in atrophy, hypopigmentation, telangiectasia, and striae formation, especially if they are used in intertriginous areas or under occlusion.
- *Pustular lesions*: Corticosteroids may precipitate pustular psoriasis, especially on withdrawal.

Preparations

- Corticosteroids are available as ointments, creams, gels, foams, and lotions:
  - Ointments are used on palms and soles.
  - Creams are used on the body.
  - Gels and lotions are used on scalp.
  - Foams (of betamethasone valerate and clobetasol propionate) are more effective than lotions and solutions used for scalp psoriasis.[16]
- Topical corticosteroids can be combined with other topical preparations such as salicylic acid, urea, lactic acid, and tar.
- They are also available as combinations with calcipotriol and tazarotene.

Topical Retinoids

History

- Retinoic acid is no longer used in the management of psoriasis.
- Topical tazarotene gel, a newer topical retinoid, has been found useful.

Mode of Action

Tazarotene has a specific retinoic acid receptor (RAR) ligand, which binds specifically to β *and* α *subtypes*, bringing down inflammation and promoting epidermal differentiation.

Use in Psoriasis

- In a gel (0.05%, 0.1%) formulation is applied once a day.
- Can also be used on face or scalp.

---

[16] Interestingly, foams have been found effective for nonscalp psoriasis as well.

- Best used in combination with Class II or III topical cortico-steroids (0.1% mometasone furoate/0.05% fluocinonide), both to improve efficacy and to minimize potential for irritation.
- Used in combination with UVB (NB) being applied prior to exposure (*c.f.* calcipotriol), but exposure of UVB is reduced by 30%.

Response

- Topical tazarotene works slower than high potency topical corticosteroids, with approximately 70% response in 3 months.
- Also reduces steroid-induced atrophy.

Side Effects

Irritation

- Burning and itching is frequent (25% of patients) and in 10% of patients, symptoms warrant withdrawal of treatment.
- Patients must be told of the potential for irritation.
- Best used in combination with topical corticosteroids, both to improve efficacy and to help minimize potential for irritation.

Preparations Available

- Tazarotene (0.05%, 0.1%) in a gel formulation
- Tazarotene + corticosteroid in a cream formulation

Newer Topical Agents

The latest topical treatments for psoriasis, including methotrexate, tapinarof, and roflumilast, represent significant advancements in disease management, targeting specific pathways involved in the condition's pathology and offering improved outcomes for patients.

Topical Methotrexate

- Earlier studies failed to show response of psoriasis to topical methotrexate.
  - Newer modes of delivery include:
    - Using penetration enhancers such as decyl methyl sulfoxide, laurocapram, propylene glycol, and isopropyl alcohol.
    - Use of microemulsion is even better than delivery from aqueous solution.

- Use of 0.25% and 1% in hydrophilic gel has been found clinically effective and well tolerated.

Tapinarof

Mode of Action

Tapinarof is a topical aryl hydrocarbon receptor-modulating agent that works through modulation of T helper type 17 (Th17) cytokines, like interleukin (IL) 17A, and IL-17F. It was approved for the treatment of plaque psoriasis in adults.

Use in Psoriasis

In a cream (1%) formulation is applied once a day to the affected area.

Response

In PSOARING 1 and PSOARING 2 trials at 12 weeks, patients in the tapinarof group were more likely to achieve a physician global assessment (PGA) score of 0 (Clear) or 1 (almost clear) than the placebo group (35.4% vs. 6%).

Side Effects

Side effects include folliculitis, contact dermatitis, and headache.

Roflumilast

Mode of Action

Roflumilast is a topical phosphodiesterase 4 inhibitor. It was approved by Food and Drug Administration (FDA) in 2022 as a topical cream for treatment of plaque psoriasis in people 12 years of age and older.

Use in Psoriasis

In a cream (0.3%) formulation is applied once a day to the affected area.

Response

In the initial randomized phase 2 trials, Roflumilast 0.3% cream was found to be more effective than placebo in patients with chronic plaque psoriasis affecting 2–20% surface area.

Side Effects

Side effects include application-site reactions and gastrointestinal side effects.

Phototherapy and Photochemotherapy

Introduction

Phototherapy is the use of nonionizing radiation for therapeutic benefit while photochemotherapy is the use of light in the presence of chemicals for the same purpose. The methods available include:
- Heliotherapy and balneophototherapy
- Broad band ultraviolet B (UVB)
- Narrow band UVB
- Lasers
- Ultraviolet A (UVA)-1
- Psoralen plus ultraviolet A (PUVA)/PUVA sol.

Heliotherapy and Balneophototherapy

- *Heliotherapy:* It is the use of sunlight in the treatment of various dermatoses because Sun is a rich source of both UVA and UVB. Since psoriasis is responsive to therapy with UVA and UVB, heliotherapy is one of the safest alternatives in the treatment of psoriasis, in the modern world of aggressive medications.
- *Balneophototherapy:* It uses saltwater bathing in combination with heliotherapy.

Dead Sea Therapy

Basis of Dead Sea Therapy

The Dead Sea is a popular location for balneophototherapy because:
- Sun shines almost constantly for 300 days in a year.
- The Dead Sea is the lowest point (>396 m below sea level) in the world, with high oxygen pressure.[1]

---

[1]Because of high atmospheric pressure.

- Even after prolonged exposure, the risk of developing sunburn is low because the sun rays falling on the Dead Sea contain mainly UVA and longer wavelengths of UVB and very little of erythemogenic short wavelength UVB because:
    - Shorter wavelengths of UVB[2] are filtered out by the atmosphere which is thick[3] and contains large amount of water vapor.
    - Shorter wavelengths of UVB are also scattered more than longer wavelength ultraviolet light (UVL).
- The Dead Sea has an average salinity of 30% and is very rich in natural minerals and other chemicals, e.g., the Dead Sea water contains about 2.3 g/L of bromine. The salts present probably have a keratolytic effect and also enhance the effect of UV radiation (UVR) on the skin.
- Rest and relaxation further contribute to the treatment success.

Response

- Recommended duration of the Dead Sea therapy is 3–4 weeks.[4]
- Two-thirds of psoriatic patients either go into remission or show excellent response and only 2% show no improvement—these are patients with resistant psoriasis such as erythroderma, pustular psoriasis, or palmoplantar psoriasis.

Broad Band Ultraviolet B Therapy

Broad band (BB) UVB is UVR with wavelength of 270–390 nm.

Treatment Protocols

- Broad band-ultraviolet B (BB-UVB) has been used in a thrice weekly schedule, after application of emollients.
- *Goeckerman's regimen:* BB-UVB therapy is used in combination with coal tar as part of Goeckerman's regimen.
- *Combination therapy:* BB-UVB is also used in combination with several other topical and systemic antipsoriatic agents such as

---

[2]*Short wavelength UVB*: It causes erythema and sunburn.
[3]The Dead Sea is the lowest point in the world.
[4]The stay of 3–4 weeks works out cheaper than hospitalization. So, the visit to the Dead Sea is a therapeutic holiday.

anthralin, calcipotriol, tazarotene, topical steroids, acitretin, and methotrexate in patients with moderate-to-severe disease.

Adverse Effects

Acute

The only significant short-term side effect is erythema.

Chronic

The important long-term side effect is photoaging.

Narrow Band Ultraviolet B Therapy

Wavelength

- The wavelength of therapeutic UVR for psoriasis is 290–320 nm with the best optimal therapeutic index[5] at 312 nm. This is because shorter wavelengths are more erythemogenic and longer wavelengths less therapeutic.
- Narrow band-ultraviolet B (NB-UVB) is UVR with wavelength of 311 ± 2 nm. It is produced by fluorescent lamps (Philips TL-01), coated with phosphor which emits UVR with a peak emission at 311 nm (± 2 nm) and a minor peak at 305 nm.

Mechanism of Action

Narrow band-ultraviolet B has immunosuppressive properties and acts in psoriasis by:
- Depleting the immunocompetent T-cells from the epidermis and dermis by inducing apoptosis[6] due to direct cytotoxic effect on the infiltrating lymphocytes.
- Suppressing the function of antigen presenting cells (Langerhans' cells) by causing photoisomerization of trans to cis-urocanic acid.
- Lowering the peripheral NK cell activity.
- Inhibiting cytokine production by both Th1 (IL-2, IFN-γ) and Th2 (IL-10) cells.

---

[5]*Optimal therapeutic dose*: It is defined as the lowest fraction of minimal erythema dose required to remit psoriatic lesions.

[6]*Apoptosis*: Programmed cell death.

It is more effective than BB-UVB because:
- Of its deeper penetration
- Higher doses (more joules/exposure) of NB-UVB can be delivered to the patient, due to its lower erythemogenic potential than BB-UVB.[7]

Side Effects

The following side effects may be encountered during NB-UVB therapy:
- *Dry skin:* Dryness and itching is not uncommon but can easily be treated with liberal use of emollients and antihistamines.
- *Acute sunburn*: Mild erythema occurs occasionally, but a burn (intense erythema, edema, or bullae formation) is rare. Burns should be treated with:
  - Application of ice packs
  - Oral nonsteroidal anti-inflammatory drugs
  - Topical steroids
  - Subsequent scheduled NBUVB treatment should be avoided and later follow the missed appointment schedules as given on page 108.
  - Adjustment of future doses of UVB.
- *Pigmentation:* Tanning and freckling occur occasionally but are less common than with PUVA therapy. Prevented by protecting uninvolved skin.
- *Folliculitis:* Use of emollients compounded by warmth and perspiration which occurs during the therapy, leads to blocking and irritation of the hair follicles.
- Long-term studies regarding development of skin cancers are not available but are probably only a remote possibility.

Use in Psoriasis

Indications

Narrow band-ultraviolet B is indicated in:
- Moderate-to-severe psoriasis involving >20% body surface area and/or Psoriasis Area and Severity Index (PASI) score of >10.
- Long standing psoriasis, not responding to conventional topical medical treatment.

---

[7]BB-UVB contains substantial amount of the more erythemogenic UV, i.e., shorter wavelengths around 290–300 nm.

- Psoriasis in patients in whom antipsoriasis drugs are contraindicated, e.g., pregnancy.

Contraindications

Narrow band-ultraviolet B should not be given in patients with:
- Photoaggravated psoriasis
- Photosensitivity disorders such as systemic lupus erythematosus, Bloom's syndrome, etc.
- History of previous cutaneous malignancies
- Unsure about attending the treatment schedule regularly

Treatment Protocols

Two protocols are followed for NB-UVB:
- Minimal erythema dose (MED)-based
- Skin phototype-based

Minimal Erythema Dose-based Protocol

- *Pretreatment assessment:*
  - A thorough medical history, physical examination, and clinical assessment of the patient, including PASI score, is necessary.
  - *Determination of MED:*[8] Prior to therapy, MED for NB-UVB is determined in each patient:
    - Determined on unaffected upper back or volar aspect of forearm (always sun protected area).
    - The test sites are irradiated with increasing doses **(Table 11.1)** of UVB (311 nm). For Indian patients, (skin types IV, V, and VI), 500, 750, 1,000, 1,200, 1,400, 1,600, 1,800, and 2,000, mJ/cm^2 is a sensitive dose ladder to determine MED.
    - Exposed sites are examined at 24 hours and the minimum dose of UVB which causes visual erythema is taken as MED. Erythema should be identifiable and within the margin of photo-tested parts.
- *Dose of NB-UVB* **(Flowchart 11.1)**: Schedule usually used for NB-UVB is a MED-based, low percentage incremental, 3–4 times

---

[8]*MED*: It is the minimum dose of UVB that produces faint uniform erythema at 24 hours.

TABLE 11.1: Dose (mJ/cm^2) of narrow band-ultraviolet B (NB-UVB) given to determine minimal erythema dose (MED).

Skin phototypes I–III	Skin phototypes IV–VI
400	500
600	750
800	1,000
1,000	1,200
1,200	1,400
1,400	1,600
	1,800
	2,000

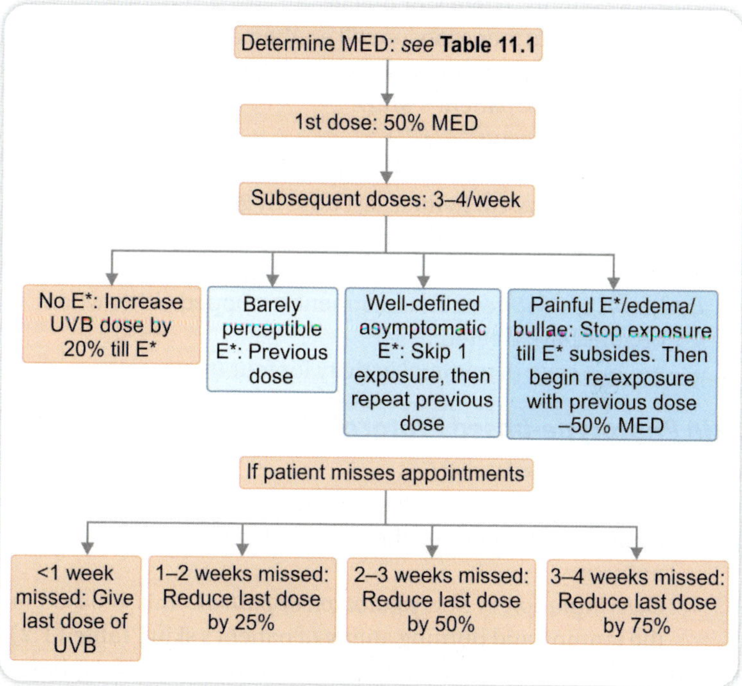

E*: Erythema

Flowchart 11.1: Minimal erythema dose (MED)-based protocol for narrow band-ultraviolet B (NB-UVB) therapy.

a week regimen. The dosage of NB-UVB should never exceed four times MED.

- *Initial dose of UVB:* 50–70% of MED. Safest to begin with 50% of MED.
- *Increments of UVB:* At each visit the dose of NB-UVB is increased, based on the erythema response to the previous dose:
  - *No erythema:* 20% increment at next visit.
  - *Grade 1 erythema* (barely perceptible erythema):
    - Repeat previous dose
  - *Grade 2 erythema* (well-defined asymptomatic erythema):
    - Skip one exposure
    - Repeat previous dose at next visit
  - *Grade 3 erythema:* Painful erythema, persisting for >24 hours, edema, or bullae:
    - No further exposure till erythema has subsided.
    - When treatment is restarted, UVB dose is reduced by 50% of patient's MED.
- *Missed appointments:*
  - *If <1 week missed:* Give the last dose of UVB.
  - *1–2 weeks missed:* Reduce last dose by 25%.
  - *2–3 weeks missed:* Reduce last dose by 50%.
  - *3–4 weeks missed:* Start from beginning.
- *End point of treatment:* The treatment is stopped either when:
  - Lesions have cleared.
  - Are in a state of minimal activity for four treatments.

Skin Phototype-based Protocol (Flowchart 11.2)

- *Pretreatment assessment:*
  - A thorough medical history, physical examination, and clinical assessment of the patient, including PASI score, is necessary.
  - *Determination of skin phototype of patient:* This is based on the tanning and burning ability of patient's skin **(Table 11.2)**.
- *Dose of NB-UVB:* Prefixed in this protocol, the dose used is based on skin color.
  - *Initial dose of UVB:* It is based on the skin phototype **(Table 11.3)**.
  - *Increments of UVB:* At each visit, the dose of NB-UVB is increased based on erythema response to the previous dose:

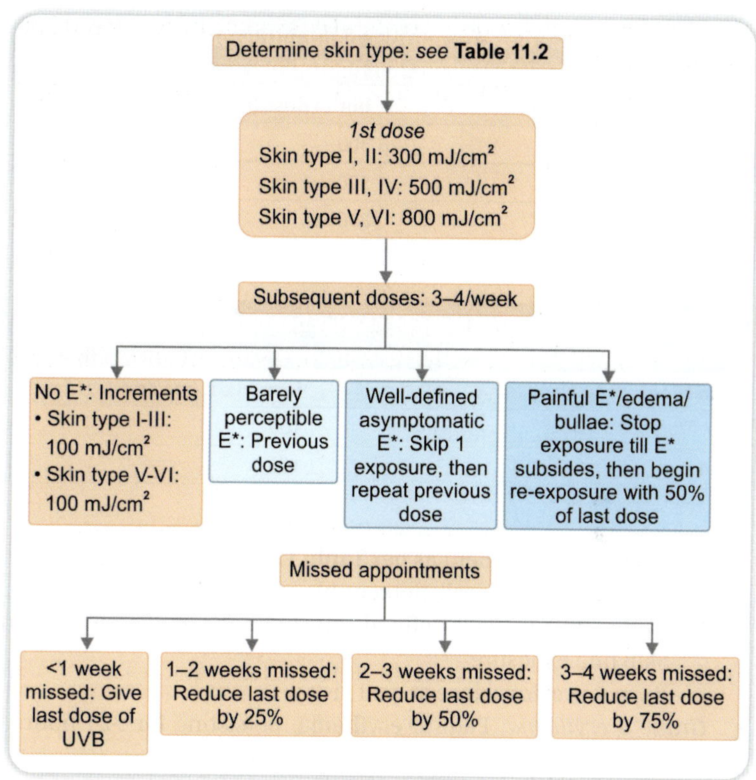

E*: Erythema

Flowchart 11.2: Skin phototype-based protocol for narrow band-ultraviolet B (NB-UVB) therapy.

TABLE 11.2: Determination of skin phototype.			
Skin phototype	**Constitutive skin color**	**Ability to burn**	**Ability to tan**
I	White	High	Very poor
II	White	High	Poor
III	White	Moderate	Good
IV	Olive	Low	Very good
V	Brown	Very low	Very good
VI	Black	Very low	Excellent

TABLE 11.3: Initial dose of narrow band-ultraviolet B (NB-UVB) for treatment of psoriasis based on skin phototype.

Skin phototype	Initial dose (mJ/cm^2)
I, II	300
III, IV	500
V, VI	800

TABLE 11.4: Increments of dose of narrow band-ultraviolet B (NB-UVB) for treatment of psoriasis based on skin phototype.

Skin type	Increment (mJ/cm^2)
I–IV	100
V–VI	150

- *No erythema:* Increment as per **Table 11.4**.
- *Grade 1 erythema* (barely perceptible erythema): Previous dose
- *Grade 2 erythema* (well-defined asymptomatic erythema):
  - Skip one exposure
  - Repeat previous dose at next visit
- *Grade 3 erythema*: Painful erythema, persisting for >24 hours, edema, or bulla:
  - No further exposures till erythema has subsided.
  - When treatment is restarted, UVB dose is reduced to half of last dose.
  - Followed by increments as mentioned in **Table 11.4**.
- *Missed appointments:* As for MED-based protocol (page 108).
- *End point of treatment:* The treatment is stopped as for the MED-based protocol.
- *The maximum dosage of NB-UVB:* Should not exceed 3,000 and 5,000 mJ in skin type IV–VI respectively.

Maintenance Therapy

If psoriasis has cleared by >95%.
- 1 exposure/week of NB-UVB for 4 weeks, keeping the dose same, as the last dose.
- 1 exposure/2 weeks of NB-UVB for 4 weeks, at 75% of highest dose of UVB.
- 1 exposure/4 weeks of NB-UVB, at 50% of highest dose of UVB.

Instructions to Patients

- Patients are advised to stop all oral and topical medications that increase cutaneous photosensitivity. Most common being: non steroidal anti-inflammatory drugs (NSAIDs), retinoids, antibiotics (sulphonamides, tetracycline, demeclocycline, quinolones), antihypertensives (ACE inhibitors, calcium channel blockers, hydrochlorothiazide) cardiovascular drugs (amiodarone), phenothiazines, etc. Newer drugs include BRAF inhibitors like vemurafenib and EGFR inhibitors.
- Adjuvant treatment is restricted to emollients (except on scalp, face and in flexures, where conventional therapy can be continued).
- Before exposure to UVB, patients are instructed to apply mineral oil, Vaseline or petrolatum to the psoriatic plaques, to reduce scattering of light. However, preparations containing salicylic acid[9] and calcipotriol[10] should be avoided.
- Eyes, breasts, genitals, and chronically photoexposed areas are protected during phototherapy unless lesions are present at these sites. Eyes are protected using UV protective goggles while breasts and genitalia are protected using a sunscreen as well as wearing garments.

Advantages

It has several advantages over PUVA therapy:
- Absence of drug-induced nausea
- No phototoxicity or photoallergic reaction
- Lesser darkening of skin
- No drug cost
- Safe for use in children and pregnant women
- Does not require posttreatment eye protection
- Low/no risk of cutaneous malignancies
- No waiting period between drug and exposure

Also has several advantages over BB-UVB therapy:
- Less frequent episodes of painful erythema and burning
- Lower risk of photocarcinogenesis

---

[9]*Salicylic acid*: It acts as a sunscreen but may even increase photosensitivity.
[10]*Calcipotriol*: It may be applied after the day's photoexposure.

- Faster resolution of skin lesions, using easy-to-administer, sub-erythemogenic doses
- Longer duration of remissions

Disadvantages

- May be less effective in thick lesions because of lower penetration, (*c.f.* PUVA therapy more effective).
- More frequent maintenance therapy (usually weekly) generally required than with PUVA (even as infrequent as monthly).

Sources of Narrow Band-Ultraviolet B

- Narrow band-ultraviolet B phototherapy chambers contain fluorescent TL-01/PL-01 tubes or compact fluorescent tubes (CFLs) as the source of irradiation and are available either as factory assembled units (Waldmann, National Biological Corporation, etc.) or can be customized at site with the cost of the chamber and lamps varying considerably between countries and brands.
- Tubes are available as Philips TL-01 series in 6'(100W), 4'(40W), and 2'(20W) and the compact fluorescent lights (CFLs) are available as Philips PL series as long (36W) and short (9W) CFLs. Some of these tubes can be used to convert BB-UVB (using FS or FSX series of Philips tubes) or UVA chambers (using F series of Philips tubes) to NB-UVB chambers.
- Longer 6' tubes are used for whole body cabinets, while 4' used for partial body exposure and the 2' tubes and CFLs used for treatment of small areas (hand and foot units for palmoplantar psoriasis and combs for scalp psoriasis). Sleek foldable home units are also available. The TL-01 lamps can be incorporated in the equipment either alone or in combination with UVA tubes. Combination chambers take longer to administer a treatment dose and so, although they provide flexibility, they may represent an unsatisfactory compromise for a busy phototherapy unit.

Home Narrow Band-Ultraviolet B

For patients who cannot travel to a phototherapy center. Hand-held devices are available for home use.

Laser Therapy

Excimer Laser

- Available as Xtrac ultra® and Xtrac velocity excimer laser.
- Emits monochromatic light at 308 nm with spot size of 3.2 cm^2 using a handheld device.
- Minimal erythema dose is determined and multiples (2–6 times) of MED delivered to site to be treated. Light delivered either in paint mode or tile mode.
- Total of 8–10 treatments given, as twice weekly exposures are adequate for clearance of plaques.
- Side effects are minimal and localized (blistering, hyperpigmentation) but data on long-term remissions unavailable.

Pulsed Dye Laser

- The Food and Drug Administration (FDA) approved for treating localized plaques of psoriasis.
- Destroy the tiny blood vessels that contribute to formation of psoriasis plaques.
- Given as 15–30-minute sessions every 3 weeks. Patient responds in 4–6 sessions.
- The commonest side effect is bruising and a small risk of scarring.

Photochemotherapy

Photochemotherapy is the therapeutic use of a combination of UVA (wavelength 320–400 nm) with a photosensitizing chemical (psoralens).

History

- History of photochemotherapy dates back to over 2000 years with discovery in Egypt of seeds of plant *Ammi majus* which grew on the banks of the river Nile.
- The usefulness of this plant in vitiligo was demonstrated as recently as 1947 by an Egyptian dermatologist, El Mofty and the active chemical was identified as methoxsalen (8-methoxypsoralen).

- Iranian dermatologist, Syed Abdol first used psoralens in the treatment of psoriasis.
- Subsequently, many others treated psoriasis with psoralens and improved the technique.
- Today, photochemotherapy is an established treatment modality in psoriasis.

Psoralens

Psoralens can be used topically (in localized lesions) or systemically (in extensive lesions). The three commonly used psoralens are:

1. 8-methoxypsoralen (8-MOP):
   - Most commonly used
   - Available in two forms:
     - Crystalline form, oxsoralen which reaches a peak level in the skin, 2 hours after oral ingestion. Absorption, less predictable. Dose is 0.6 mg/kg/day.
     - Encapsulated liquid form, oxsoralen ultra reaches peak level in the skin 1 hour after oral ingestion. Absorption is more predictable. Dose is 0.4 mg/kg/day.
       - Absorption is delayed and reduced by fat-rich food.
2. 5-methoxypsoralen (5-MOP):
   - Absorption only 25% that of 8-MOP; low absorption compensated by increasing dose to 1.2–1.5 mg/kg/day
   - Causes dark pigmentation
   - Requires greater cumulative dose of UVA
   - Lower gastrointestinal side effects
3. Trimethylpsoralen (TMP):
   - Mainly used for topical or bath PUVA
   - Not used orally because poorly absorbed

Source of Ultraviolet A

Action spectrum for erythema with 8-MOP, which was earlier considered to be 365 nm, has recently been shown to be around 300 nm. The sources of UVA include:

- *Artificial sources:* Most frequently used sources of UVA radiation, for therapeutic purposes, are fluorescent tubes with a peak emission at around 355 nm. Several UVA phototherapy units are available.

- Ultraviolet A photochemotherapy chambers contain fluorescent UVA tubes/CFLs as the source of irradiation and are available either as factory assembled units (Waldmann, National Biological Corporation, etc.) or can be customized at site with the cost of the chamber and lamps varying considerably between countries and brands.
  - Tubes are available as Philips F series in 6' (80–100 W), 4' (40 W), and 2' (20 W) and the CFLs are available as Philips PL series as long (36 W) and short (9 W) CFLs. Some of these tubes can be used to convert BB UVB (using FS or FSX series of Philips tubes) to UVA chambers.
  - Longer 6' tubes are used for whole body cabinets, while 4' used for partial body exposure and the 2' tubes and CFLs used for treatment of small areas (hand and foot units for palmoplantar psoriasis and combs for scalp psoriasis). Sleek foldable home units are also available. The UVA lamps can be incorporated in the chamber either alone or in combination with TL-01 tubes emitting NB-UVB.
- *Natural source:* Sunlight is an ecofriendly, inexhaustible source of UV energy. Though frequently used in conjunction with psoralens for treatment of vitiligo (PUVA sol), sunlight is now also being increasingly used as a source of UVA for treatment of psoriasis.

The amount of UVA reaching the Earth from Sun is 100–500 times that of UVB, because of greater scattering of UVB (shorter wavelengths) Though the amount of UVA in solar radiation is more constant than UVB, it depends on certain factors:

- It is more in summer than in winter.
- It is more in the tropics than in temperate areas.
- It is maximum between 1,100–1,300 hours (i.e., at noon, when the Sun is directly overhead).
- Though the amount of solar UVA reaching the earth is less on a cloudy day, there is still an adequate amount present for the patient to continue his treatment.
- Ordinary window glass does not cut off UVA (though it filters out UVB), so patient can expose through clear (also importantly clean) unbeveled large-sized window glass.

Mechanism of Action

Psoralens act in psoriasis by:

- *Effects on deoxyribonucleic acid (DNA):* Psoralens have two effects on DNA:
  - *Type I reaction:* It involves an oxygen-independent mechanism which results in formation of DNA photoadducts. Psoralens intercalate between DNA base pairs in the absence of UV radiation and induce a 2-step photochemical reaction:
    - With 1st UVA exposure, photons of UVA are absorbed and monofunctional adducts are formed with thymine and cytosine.
    - With 2nd UVA exposure, photons of UVA are absorbed and bifunctional adducts are formed, with a 5,6 double bond of the pyrimidine base of the opposite strand, producing an inter strand crosslink of DNA double helix, decreasing DNA proliferation.
  - *Type 2 reaction:* It involves an oxygen-dependent (photochemical) mechanism in which free oxygen radicals are formed. In photosensitized skin, psoralens react with free oxygen to form reactive species, causing damage to DNA. Antigen-presenting cells and T-cells are most susceptible to oxygen dependent reactions.
- *Immunosuppressive actions:* Of psoralens include:
  - Changing expression of cytokines and their receptors
  - Reducing the number of Langerhans cells and human leukocyte antigens (HLAs)

Side Effects

Acute Side Effects

- *Gastrointestinal reactions:* Anorexia, nausea, and vomiting are universal (almost). Reduced by giving medication after food, splitting the dose, using antiemetics such as domperidone and if all these measures fail then by reducing the dose.
- *Neuropsychiatric reactions:* Headache, dizziness, light headedness, depression, and insomnia are not uncommon but decrease in most patients even on continuation of therapy.

- *Cutaneous reactions*: Phototoxic reactions (which manifest as pruritus, pain, excessive erythema, and blisters). These are reduced by correct dosimetry as well as protecting the skin from inadvertent sun exposure using broad spectrum sunscreens. Other side effects include maculopapular rashes, photo-onycholysis, friction blisters, hypertrichosis, and urticaria.
- *Other side effects*: Exacerbation of asthma, fever.

Chronic Side Effects

- Cataract and transient visual field defects. UV protective goggles should be used by patients during exposure within the treatment cabin as well as when outdoors on the day of ingestion of oral psoralens. PUVA operators are also advised to wear goggles when they enter the cabin, but this is not required for any stray radiation outside the cabin.
- Cutaneous aging
- Nonmelanoma skin cancers.

Availability

Psoralens

- *8-methoxypsoralen:* Available in two forms.
    i. Oxsoralen (crystalline form) given in a dose of 0.6 mg/kg
    ii. Oxsoralen ultra (liquid form) given in a dose of 0.4 mg/kg
- *5-methoxypsoralen:* Given in a dose of 1.2–1.5 mg/kg
- Topical trimethylpsoralen

Use in Psoriasis

Indications

Psoralen plus ultraviolet A is indicated in:
- Severe, extensive psoriasis (>20% BSA[11] or PASI[12] score >10)
- Localized pustular psoriasis
- Persistent palmoplantar pustulosis
- Failure of topical treatment

---

[11]*BSA*: Body surface area.
[12]*PASI*: This is one of the standard methods of assessing the severity of psoriasis **(Annexure 3)**.

Contraindications

Systemic PUVA is absolutely contraindicated in the following:
- Pregnant and lactating women
- Children < 12 years
- Patients with xeroderma pigmentosum
- Patients with history of multiple skin cancers
- Patients who have previously been treated with ionizing radiation or with arsenic
- Patients with history of unspecified and drug photosensitivity

Systemic PUVA is preferably avoided in patients with:
- Family history of skin cancer(s)
- Collagen vascular diseases and autoimmune diseases
- Cataract
- Cardiovascular impairment

Systemic Psoralen Plus Ultraviolet A

Pretreatment Evaluation

- A comprehensive history is taken. Rule out xeroderma pigmentosum, history of cutaneous malignancies in self or family, history of having received radiation in past, and whether on photosensitizing drugs.
- Clinical examination, including ophthalmological evaluation for cataract should be carried out.
- Initial dose of UVA and its increments are based either on:
  - *Patient's skin phototype:* In American protocol, before starting PUVA therapy, patient's skin type is determined (**Table 11.2**, page 109).
  - *Minimum phototoxic dose (MPD):* In European protocol, before starting PUVA therapy, patient's MPD is determined:
    - Patient is given appropriate dose (0.4 mg/kg of liquid form or 0.6 mg/kg of crystalline form) of 8-MOP.
    - 2 hours later, a template (consisting of 6–8 fenestrations of at least 1 cm^2) is placed on the patient's buttocks or back. The skin is exposed to geometrically increasing doses of UVA, beginning with 0.5 J/cm^2 for skin type I and II and 1.5 J/cm^2 for skin types III–VI, through fenestrations of the template.
    - The MPD is the lowest dose of UVA that produces pink erythema with distinct borders, 72 hours after exposure.

Protocol for Systemic Psoralen Plus Ultraviolet A

Psoralen plus ultraviolet A treatment consists of two phases:
- *Clearing phase:* Aimed at attaining remission of psoriasis
- *Maintenance phase:* Aimed at maintaining remission

There are three protocols for treatment of psoriasis using photochemotherapy:
- *American protocol* (**Flowchart 11.3**): American protocol, based on patient's skin phototype is more frequently followed:
  - *Clearing phase:*
    - Either a twice or thrice a week schedule is followed (never on two consecutive days).

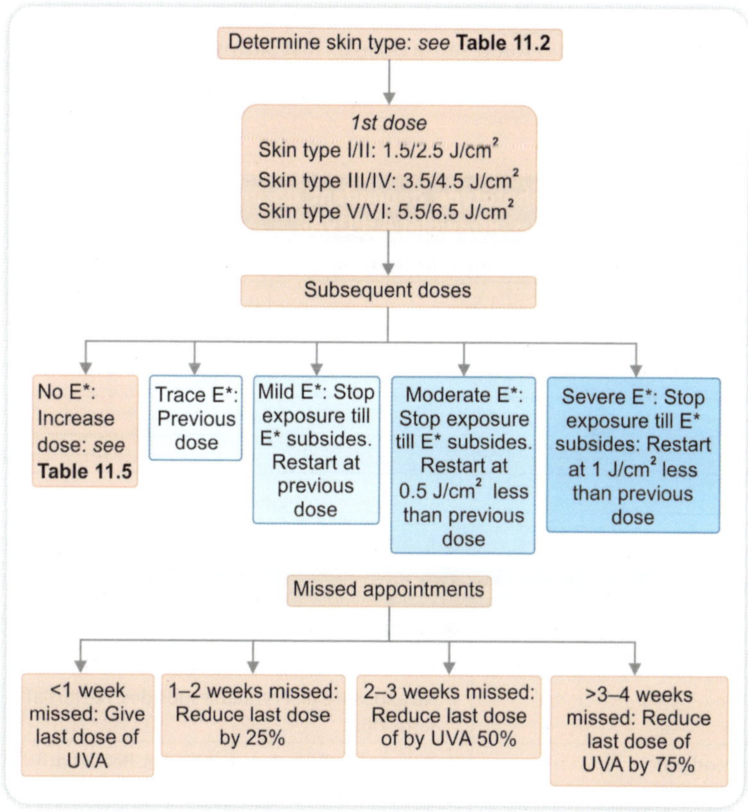

Flowchart 11.3: Skin phototype-based protocol for psoralen plus ultraviolet A (PUVA) therapy.

- 8-MOP is given in a dose of 0.4 mg/kg (liquid form) or 0.6 mg/kg (crystallized form), 1–2 hours before exposure to UVA.
    - Initial dose of UVA depending on the skin phototype **(Table 11.5)**.
    - Ultraviolet A doses are increased **(Table 11.6)** till erythema develops.
    - Next dose is decided by the amount of erythema produced by preceding exposure **(Flowchart 11.3)**.
    - Usually, 20–25 treatments are required to induce remission during clearing phase with a mean cumulative UVA dose of 80–100 J/cm^2.
  - *Missed appointments:* If the appointments have been missed for:
    - <1 week: Keep same dose as last sitting
    - 1–2 weeks: Reduce last dose by 25%

TABLE 11.5: Skin phototype dependent dosimetry of ultraviolet A (UVA) in psoralen plus ultraviolet A (PUVA).

Skin phototype	Initial dose (J/ cm^2)	Increments/week (J/cm^2)
I	1.5	0.25
II	2.5	0.5
III	3.5	0.5–1.0
IV	4.5	1.0
V	5.5	1.0
VI	6.5	1.0–1.5

TABLE 11.6: Dose of ultraviolet A (UVA) after development of erythema.

Erythema	Dose of UVA at next sitting
Trace mild	• Same dose as at previous sitting • No exposure till erythema subsides. Restart at same dose
Moderate	No exposure till erythema subsides. Restart at dose 0.5 J/cm^2 less than previous dose
Severe	No exposure till erythema subsides. Restart at dose 1 J/cm^2 less than previous dose

- 2–3 weeks: Reduce last dose by 50%
- >3 weeks: Start from initial dose
  ○ *Maintenance phase:*
    - 1 exposure/week for 4 weeks, keeping the dose same as the last dose of clearing phase.
    - 1 exposure/2 weeks for 4 weeks, decreasing the dose by 25% of last dose of clearing phase.
    - 1 exposure/4 weeks for 4 weeks, decreasing the dose by 50% of the last dose of clearing phase.
- European protocol **(Flowchart 11.4)**:
  ○ In European protocol treatments are given four times/week **(Table 11.7)**.
  ○ Initial dose is 70% of MPD (Page 118).

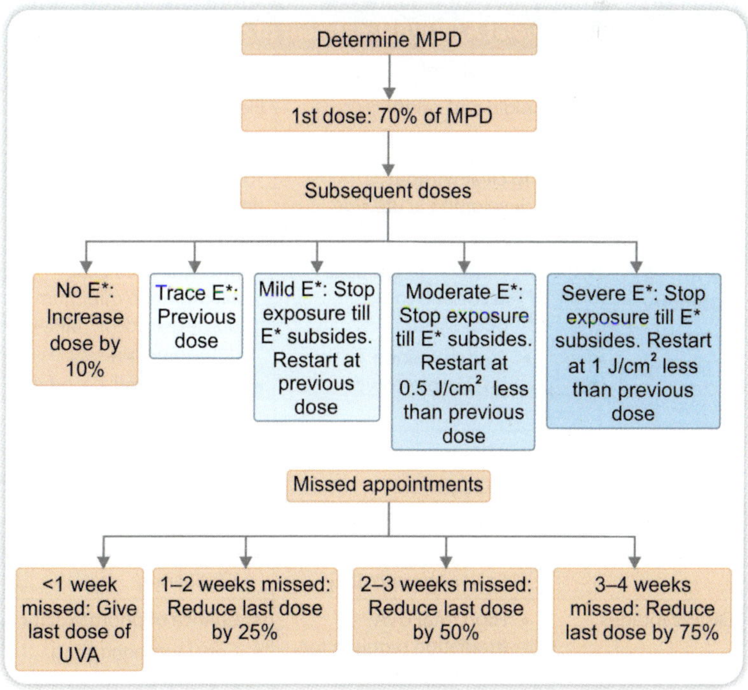

E*: Erythema

Flowchart 11.4: Minimum phototoxic dose (MPD)-based protocol for psoralen plus ultraviolet A (PUVA) therapy.

(MPD: minimum phototoxic dose)

- ○ Increments are based on the degree of erythema. Increments of 10% are given at each visit till the required erythema is achieved.
- *Psoralen plus ultraviolet A sol:* Frequently used treatment in resource poor tropical[13] settings. Though there is no standard protocol for treating patients with PUVA sol, the most frequently followed schedule includes **(Flowchart 11.5)**:
  - ○ *Clearing phase:*
- Appropriate dose of psoralens is ingested by the patient, on alternate days and emollient applied to skin.
- Lesions are exposed to direct sunlight 2–2½ hours later, starting with an initial exposure time of 5 minutes. Preferable timing for

TABLE 11.7: Differences between US and European protocols for psoralen plus ultraviolet A (PUVA) treatment of psoriasis.

	US protocol	European protocol
Approach	Rigid and careful	Flexible and aggressive
Goal	To clear without developing acute side effects	To clear rapidly without developing pigmentation
Ultraviolet A (UVA) dosimetry: • Initial • Increments	• Predetermined dose according to skin phototype • Predetermined, based on skin phototype	• Individualized dose according to minimum phototoxic dose (MPD) determination • Individualized, based on erythema
Treatments given/week	2–3 times	4 times
Advantages	• Easier to perform as doses predetermined • Lower phototoxicity	• Lower cumulative • UVA radiation required for clearing
Disadvantages	• High total UVA irradiation required for clearing • Greater pigmentation	• Chance of phototoxicity • Constant monitoring required

---

[13]*Tropical*: Because of abundance of sunlight.

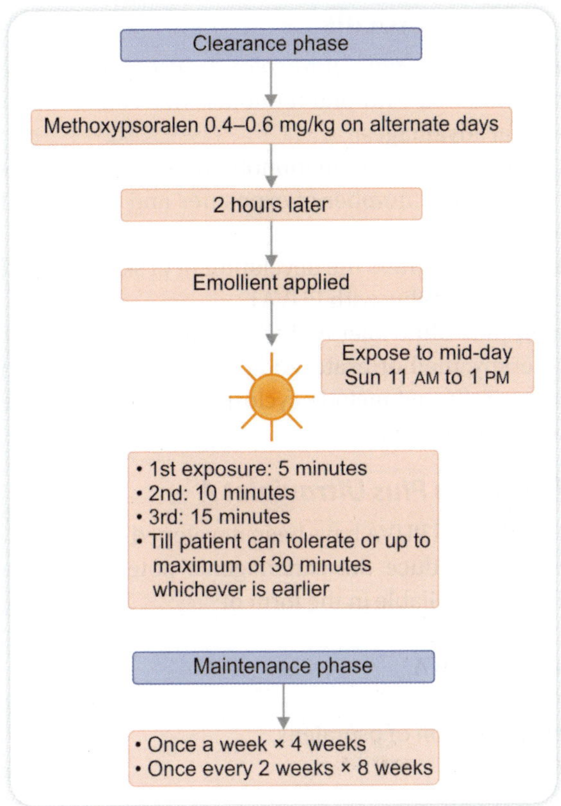

Flowchart 11.5: Protocol for systemic psoralen plus ultraviolet A (PUVA) sol.

exposure to solar radiation is between 1,100 and 1,300 hours (noon).

- Time of exposure is increased by 5 minutes every exposure until the patient can tolerate (symptoms develop) or up to a maximum of 30 minutes, whichever is earlier.
- Treatment is continued till clearance.
- *Maintenance phase*: Various schedules have been suggested:
  - Once/week for 4 weeks
  - Once every 2 weeks for 8 weeks

Combination Protocols

- *Retinoid psoralen plus ultraviolet A (RePUVA):* PUVA therapy can be combined with oral retinoids. This combination therapy has several advantages:
  - It is more effective than monotherapy with either agent.
  - It reduces the number of exposures and so cumulative UVA dose.
  - Retinoids suppress the development of skin cancers (thought to be a possibility with PUVA).
- Psoralen plus ultraviolet A (PUVA) can also be combined with UVB therapy, methotrexate, and calcipotriol. Combinations that are contraindicated include cyclosporine and PUVA, because of carcinogenic potential.

Topical Psoralen Plus Ultraviolet A

Protocols for topical PUVA have been developed to limit the systemic side effects and reduce the carcinogenic potential of oral PUVA. Topical PUVA is available in the form of:
- Bath water PUVA
- Bathing suit PUVA
- PUVA soak therapy
- Direct application of psoralens
- PUVA comb

Bath Water Psoralen Plus Ultraviolet A

- The efficacy of bath PUVA therapy is almost similar to oral PUVA, so it is an effective alternative.
- Patient soaks himself (except for the head) in a dilute solution of psoralen in a bathtub for 15 minutes, dries off and then immediately irradiates with UVA in a conventional phototherapy unit. Patient should wash himself thoroughly with soap and water after UV irradiation.
- *Preparation of psoralen bath:*
  - *Trimethylpsoralen bath*: 100 mL of TMP stock solution containing 0.05% (0.5 mg/mL) TMP in ethanol is added to 150 L of water at 37–38°C to give a solution with a concentration of 0.3 mg/L.

- ○ *8-MOP bath*: 50 mL of 0.75% alcoholic solution of 8-MOP (commercially available in India) is diluted in 100 L of water to give a final concentration of 3.75 mg/L.
- *Treatment protocol* (**Flowchart 11.6**):
  - ○ *Schedule*: Treatment is given 3–5 days a week.
  - ○ *Starting dose*: MPD is determined on untanned buttock after a psoralen bath and an initial dose of 30–50% of MPD is recommended (usually around 0.5 J/cm^2) for all skin types.
  - ○ *Increment schedule and final dose*: It depends on the psoralen used:
    - – With 8-MOP bath, weekly increments of 0.1–0.2 J/cm^2 up to a UVA dose of 1.0-1.5 J/cm^2 and then increments

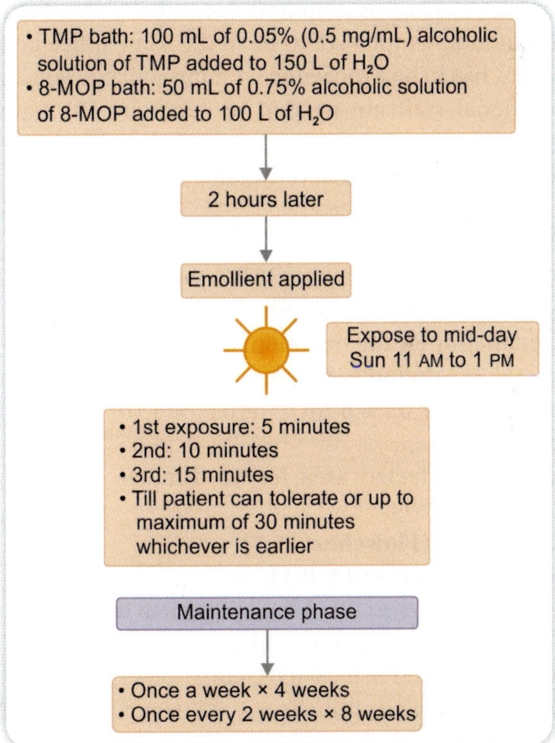

Flowchart 11.6: Protocol for bath psoralen plus ultraviolet A (PUVA) therapy.

(MOP: 8-methoxypsoralen; TMP: trimethylpsoralen)

are increased to 0.5–1.0 J/cm² up to a dose of 12 J/cm² (erythema threshold).
- With TMP bath, weekly increments of 0.1–0.2 J/cm² up to a UVA dose of 1–2 J/cm²
  ○ *Maintenance treatment*: Given to maintain remissions:
    - Once or twice a week for 1–2 months is generally recommended.
    - Patients with frequent relapses can be given long-term therapy once every 1–2 weeks.
    - If relapse occurs during maintenance, the patient is restarted on the clearing schedule.
- *Disadvantages:* Providing bathing facilities have their own economic, logistical, and sanitary implications:
  ○ Adequate space is required since both the bathtub and phototherapy unit have to be in the same office because the patient has to be exposed to UVA immediately after soaking.
  ○ Additional staff are needed to supervise the bathing and therapy.
  ○ Providing cleanliness and hygiene.

Soak Psoralen Plus Ultraviolet A Therapy

- It is a modified version of bath PUVA therapy.
- Both 8-MOP and TMP are used.
- It is used mainly for the treatment of hands and feet.
- The psoralen solution is prepared by adding 6 mL of alcoholic solution of either 0.1% 8-MOP or 0.05% TMP to 10 L of hot tap water at 42–45°C.
  Patient soaks affected area for 15 minutes and immediately exposes to UVA rays.
- *With TMP soaks* (**Flowchart 11.7**):
  ○ *Initial dose of UVA:* 0.1–0.4 J/cm²
  ○ *Weekly increments:* 0.1–0.2 J/cm² up to a dose of 5 J/cm²
- *With 8-MOP soaks* (**Flowchart 11.7**):
  ○ *Initial dose of UVA:* 0.25–0.8 J/cm²
  ○ *Weekly increment:* Initially 0.1–0.2 J/cm² up to a UVA dose of 1 J/cm² and then weekly increment of 0.3–0.5 J/cm² depending on the response, up to a dose of 12 J/cm².

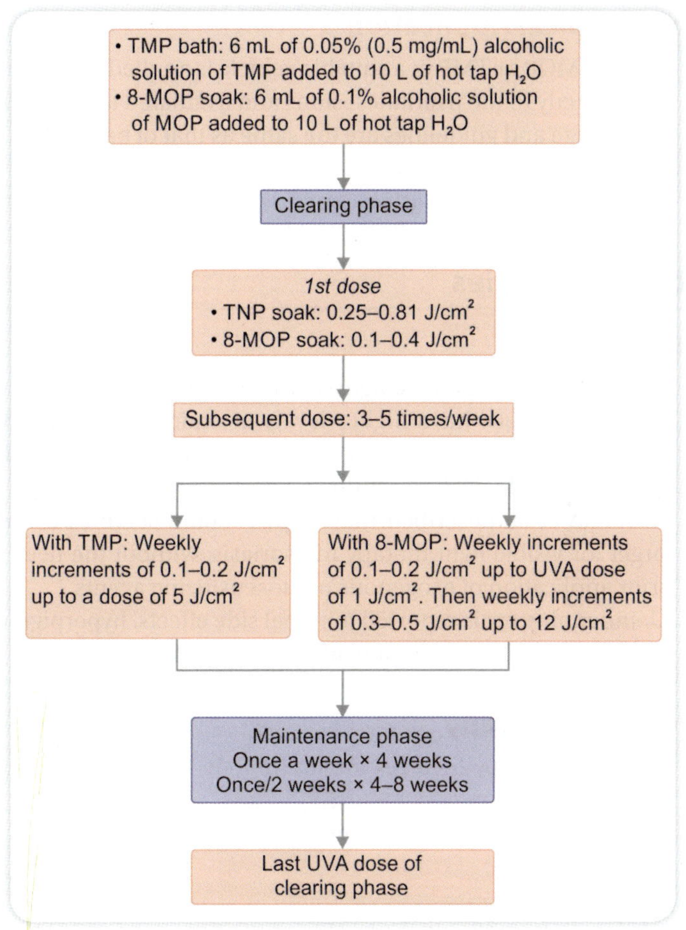

Flowchart 11.7: Protocol for soak psoralen plus ultraviolet A (PUVA) therapy.

(MOP: 8-methoxypsoralen; TMP: trimethylpsoralen)

- Patient washes his hands and feet with soap and water after UVA exposure.
- *Maintenance treatment:*
  - Maintenance dose is usually at the last UVA dose of the clearing phase.
  - Given once a week for 4 weeks followed by once in 2 weeks for a period of 4–8 weeks.

Direct Topical Application

- Either 8-MOP or TMP in a suitable vehicle is applied on alternate days directly to the psoriatic lesions and irradiated after 1 hour.
- The dosage and guidelines are the same as that of bath PUVA.
- *Indications*:
  - Palmoplantar psoriasis/pustulosis

Other Modalities

Visible Light

- Visible light (blue and red light) has been tried to treat psoriasis.
- Psoriatic plaques have higher levels of endogenous protoporphyrin IX (PpIX) than normal-appearing skin or skin affected by other dermatologic diseases do.
- Bisonette et al. described that "PpIX" could serve as a viable target for visible light therapy in psoriasis, without the need for prior application of exogenous photosensitizing agents.
- Kleinpenning et al. reported minimal side effects, hyperpigmentation was the most common adverse effect noticed.

Grenz Ray Therapy

- Grenz ray therapy involves the use of long-wavelength ionizing radiation.
- Historically used, rarely used now.

Systemic Therapy

Introduction

Systemic therapy in psoriasis is indicated in:
- Extensive disease [body surface area (BSA) > 10%; Psoriasis Area and Severity Index (PASI) > 10]
- Recalcitrant palmoplantar disease impacting patient's quality of life
- Localized lesions not responding to topical therapy

The systemic drugs used in psoriasis include:
- Methotrexate (Mtx)
- Cyclosporin A (CsA)
- Acitretin
- Hydroxyurea
- Biologics
- Phosphodiesterase inhibitors
- Janus kinase inhibitors
- Other investigational drugs

Systemic therapy is invariably combined with topical therapy and sometimes even the systemic drugs are used in combination, either simultaneously or sequentially.

Methotrexate

History

- In 1950s, used for treating leukemia
- In 1960s, found to be effective in psoriasis
- In 1964, Van Scott et al. first used weekly doses of Mtx intramuscularly for treating psoriasis.

- In 1969, oral weekly dose used for first time
- In 1971, Weinstein and Frost used Mtx in a weekly schedule of three divided doses. In the same year it was approved by Food and Drug Administration (FDA) for use in severe psoriasis.

Mechanism of Action

In psoriasis, Mtx acts by:
- Immunosuppressive action—Mtx:
  - Induces T-cell apoptosis.
  - Shifts the TH1 response to TH2 response.
- *Antichemotactic action*: Mtx reduces neutrophilic and mono-nuclear cell chemotaxis.
- *Antimitotic action*: Mtx inhibits enzyme dihydrofolate reductase and so reduces epidermal cell proliferation.

Pharmacokinetics

- *Absorption*: In psoriatics, the intestinal absorption is variable, but on an average about 70% is absorbed. In children, absorption decreases in the presence of milk and food but not in adults. Doses more than 25 mg is preferably given parenterally because of erratic gut absorption.
- *Circulation*: 70% circulates bound to plasma albumin.
- *Excretion*: 95% excreted by kidney.
- *Drug interactions*: To avoid toxicity of Mtx, concomitant use of certain drugs should be avoided:
  - Drugs which increase serum level[1] of Mtx by displacing it from plasma protein binding, e.g., sulfonamides, salicylates, phenytoin, and barbiturates.
  - Drugs which increase serum levels of Mtx by decreasing its renal elimination, e.g., frusemide and probenecid.
  - Drugs which have similar side effect toxicity profile, e.g., corticosteroids (like Mtx) are immunosuppressive and can also cause peptic ulceration.

Side Effects and Management

At a dose of 15–22.5 mg weekly, side effects though uncommon may occasionally be seen.

---

[1]*Increase the serum level*: Thereby increasing its toxicity.

General

- Many patients complain of fatigue and a feeling of being unwell for 24 hours after weekly dose.
- Patients receiving high parenteral doses, often complain of headache (often bursting) and dizziness.
- Fever is less common.

Gastrointestinal System

- Include nausea, anorexia, diarrhea, vomiting, stomatitis, and mucosal erosions.
- Of these, nausea and vomiting are frequently troublesome initially, but subside with continued use. If they persist, symptoms reduced by:
  - Adding 5 mg folic acid[2] weekly
  - Taking the drug after food or splitting the dose of Mtx
  - Taking domperidone half an hour before Mtx if nausea is severe.

Hematological Side Effects

- Develop with Mtx overdosage (e.g., if patient takes drug daily), if patient is dehydrated, in patients with declining renal function and those on other folate reductase inhibitors (cotrimoxazole).
- Maximal myelosuppression occurs 7–10 days after oral dose.
- Manifest as folate deficient megaloblastic anemia, thrombocytopenia, leucopenia, and pancytopenia.
- In case of acute overdosage/toxicity, leucovorin calcium (folinic acid or citrovorum factor) is used as an antidote (leucovorin rescue).
  - Administered immediately[3] in a dose of 20 mg (10 mg/m^2) parenterally and repeated every 6 hours, either orally or parenterally.[4]
  - If blood levels of Mtx can be measured, this should be done every 12–24 hours and dose of leucovorin adjusted till Mtx level falls below 10^{-8} M:

---

[2]*Folic acid*: Recent evidence suggests that high (5 mg/day) doses of folic acid may reduce efficacy of methotrexate and many dermatologists therefore now prescribe 1 mg/day or 5 mg/week of folic acid, instead of 5 mg daily.
[3]Within 24–36 hours.
[4]Doses of leucovorin of >25 mg given parenterally.

  - If serum Mtx level is 0.5×10^{-6} M, leucovorin dose is 20 mg, 6 hourly.
  - If serum Mtx level is 0.1×10^{-5} M leucovorin dose is 100 mg, 6 hourly.
  - If serum Mtx level is 0.2×10^{-5} M, leucovorin dose is 200 mg, 6 hourly.
- In case of massive overdose, hydration and alkalinization is needed to prevent precipitation of Mtx and its metabolites in renal tubules.
- Further treatment with Mtx is withheld, till toxicity settles down.

Hepatotoxicity

Hepatotoxicity is a major side-effect of Mtx:
- Presents as transaminitis (frequently) and hepatitis, fibrosis, and cirrhosis (less frequently). The clinical course of cirrhosis induced by Mtx is probably not aggressive.
- The potential for liver toxicity increases in presence of diabetes, in obese patients, alcoholics, and in patients with preexisting liver disease.

Cutaneous Side Effects

Cutaneous adverse effects include:
- Burning sensation of psoriatic plaques, lasting several days and heralds rapid resolution of lesions. Pruritus, pain, and ulceration of the psoriatic plaques can occur. Mtx induced skin necrosis has also been reported. Treated with emollients.
- Rarely, metastasizing squamous cell carcinoma with a relative risk of 2:1 in patients who have received large doses (3 g) over long periods of time (4 years). This risk is independent of the use of psoralen with ultraviolet A (PUVA).

Reproductive Adverse Effects

- Methotrexate is a teratogenic and mutagenic. Pregnancy and impregnation should be avoided while on treatment and for 1 (for females)-3 (for males) months thereafter.
- Causes oligospermia, and so avoided in men who have not completed their family.

Rare Side Effects

- *Pulmonary*: Rarely causes life-threatening (15% mortality) acute interstitial pneumonitis due to hypersensitivity reaction. Patients present with dry cough and breathlessness and fibrosis.
- *Central nervous system*: Acute depression
- *Methotrexate osteopathy*:
  - Seen in patients on low-dose therapy for long periods of time.
  - Presents with triad of severe pain, osteoporosis, and compression fractures localized to lower end of tibia.
  - Responds to withdrawal of Mtx.

Use in Psoriasis

The decision to use Mtx in psoriasis is individualized and is influenced by:

- Degree of severity, based on extent and type of involvement
- Discomfort caused to the patient, including its effect on patient's quality of life
- Whether jeopardizing economic activity
- Psychological condition of the patient

Indications

Methotrexate is indicated in:

- Extensive psoriasis (including erythrodermic) involving >20% of BSA.
- Moderately severe psoriasis, not responding to conventional therapy.
- Psoriasis of certain areas affecting the normal function of patient, e.g., psoriasis of palms and soles.
- Generalized pustular psoriasis
- Localized pustular psoriasis of specific sites, e.g., of palms and soles
- Psoriatic arthropathy

Contraindications

Methotrexate is *absolutely contraindicated* in:

- Pregnant and lactating women
- Patients with active hepatitis

- Patients with cirrhosis of liver, with compromise of liver function
- HIV-positive patients
- Patients with active peptic ulcer and ulcerative colitis

Methotrexate is *preferably avoided* in patients:
- With abnormal liver function tests (LFTs)
- With hepatitis B and C infection
- With abnormal renal function tests
- With leucopenia and thrombocytopenia
- Who are obese or who have diabetes mellitus, because of increased potential for hepatotoxicity
- In reproductive age group, because of teratogenic and mutagenic potential
- Who consume excessive amounts of alcohol
- Who are elderly, because of reduced renal clearance and so are more prone to developing pancytopenia
- Who are unreliable, as they may continue to take the drug even when asked to stop

Treatment Protocols

Dose

- *Dose*: 0.2–0.4 mg/kg/week, up to a maximum of 0.5 mg/kg. However, dose should not exceed 30 mg/week. A dose of >25 mg is preferably given parenterally.
- *Test dose*:[5] If the baseline investigations are normal:
  - Test dose of 2.5–5 mg of Mtx is given orally.
  - Hemogram and LFTs are done 7–10 days after test dose to detect any idiosyncratic reactions.
- *Full dose*: If repeat investigations are within the normal limits, then the full dose (7.5–22.5 mg) is given as either:
  - Single dose, given weekly
  - Or three divided doses, administered at 12 hourly intervals, given at weekly intervals.
- Both, the single and divided dose therapy are equally effective. Always add folic acid, 5 mg weekly when patient is on Mtx.

---

[5]*Test dose*: Many dermatologists do away with giving a test dose.

Duration of Treatment

- Methotrexate is continued till there is 80–90% improvement.[6]
- It is then either stopped abruptly or tapered by 2.5–5 mg every 1–2 weeks.

Adjuvant Therapy

Conventional topical therapy (emollients) is continued during Mtx therapy and even thereafter.

Variations in Treatment Protocol

- *Parenteral administration*: It can be administered parenterally either as an intramuscular or intravenous bolus dose in patients who do not respond to oral Mtx.[7] Such patients may improve rapidly with parenteral Mtx. Parenteral therapy is also preferred, if dose >25 mg.
- *In elderly*: Lower weekly dose of 7.5 mg is recommended and if the patient's disease warrants a higher dose, the patient should be carefully monitored by more frequent hemogram and renal and LFTs.
- *Combination therapy*: Mtx can be combined with other topical or systemic therapies to achieve a better response and to reduce its side effects. Though Mtx is often combined with several systemic agents, it is important to remember that with:
  - *PUVA/PUVA sol and narrow band UVB (NB-UVB):* There is a debatable increase in incidence of cutaneous malignancies.
  - *Cyclosporin:* There may be severe immunosuppression.
  - *Retinoids:* There may be increased hepatotoxicity.
- *Rotational therapy*: To reduce side effects and to decrease the cumulative dose of a single drug, rotational therapy is frequently employed. Drugs used in rotational treatment along with Mtx are:
  - PUVA/PUVA sol
  - Cyclosporin
  - Retinoids
  - Hydroxyurea
- *In relapsed psoriasis*: In cases of relapse involving more than 20% BSA, Mtx can be restarted without the test dose.

---

[6]With methotrexate, it is just not necessary to continue medication till 100% improvement.

[7]Because intestinal absorption of methotrexate in patients with psoriasis is erratic.

Monitoring Patients on Methotrexate (Flowchart 12.1)

Pretreatment Evaluation

Before starting Mtx, the following investigations are mandatory:

- Complete hemogram, because it is myelotoxic. Rule out macrocytosis.
- LFTs, because it is hepatotoxic.
- Renal function tests, because it is excreted through kidney.
- Chest X-ray (CXR), to rule out any infection because it is immunosuppressive and because rarely Mtx causes interstitial pneumonitis.
- Serological screening for hepatitis B and C and HIV in high-risk patients.
- Pre-Mtx liver biopsy is not routinely done but is indicated in patients with history of following risk factors:
  - Liver disease, including hepatitis B and C infection
  - Diabetes
  - Obesity
  - Alcohol intake
  - Intravenous drug use.

Follow-up Evaluations

Careful monitoring of patient during Mtx therapy is necessary to look for:

- *Hematological evaluation*: Complete hemogram repeated (2–3 days prior to scheduled next dose) every 2 weeks for 8 weeks and then every 4–8 weeks.
  - If hematological parameters remain normal, then Mtx is continued till necessary.
  - If hemoglobin falls below 7 g%, platelets below 100,000/mm^3, or total leukocyte count below 4,000/mm^3, Mtx is discontinued for 2 weeks and hemogram repeated.
    - If reports are normal, Mtx reinstituted.
    - If reports are still abnormal, institute alternative therapy.
- *Hepatic evaluation:*
  - LFTs: These are repeated every 2 weeks for 4 weeks and then 4 weekly. If transaminases are elevated more than three times, Mtx is discontinued for 2 weeks and LFTs is repeated.

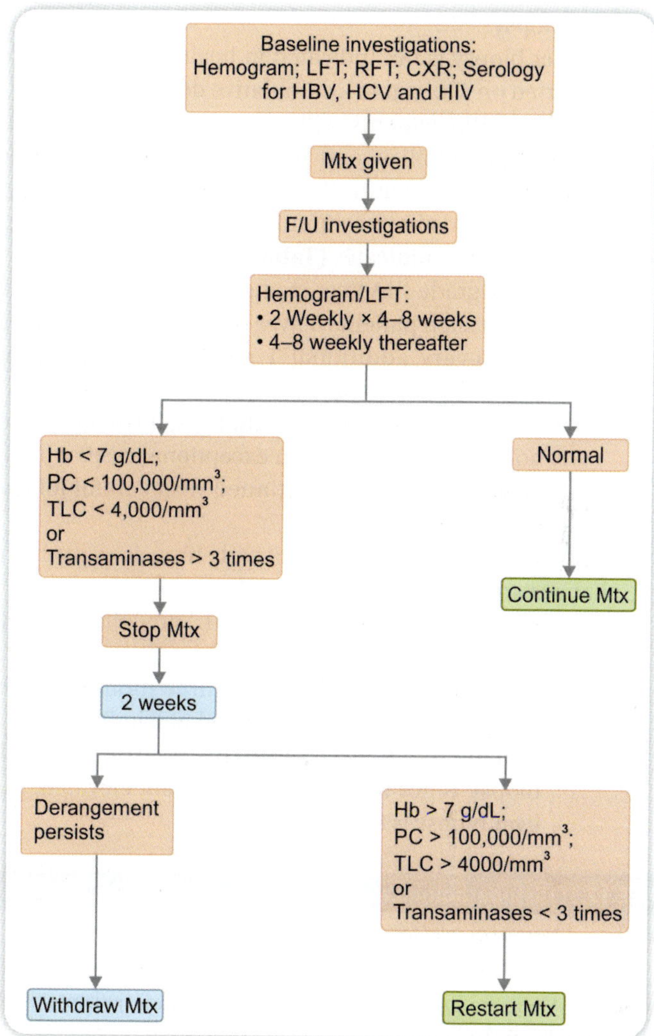

Flowchart 12.1: Algorithm for monitoring patients on methotrexate.

(CXR: chest X-ray; F/U: follow-up; Hb: hemoglobin; HBV: hepatitis B virus; HCV: hepatitis C virus; HIV: human immunodeficiency virus; LFT: liver function test; Mtx: methotrexate; PC: platelet count; RFT: renal function test; TLC: total leukocyte count)

- If transaminase levels have returned to normal, Mtx can be restarted.
- If transaminases continue to be elevated, then alternate therapy is instituted.

- ○ Liver biopsy:
  - – Liver biopsy is not indicated in healthy individuals to be started on Mtx (up to a cumulative dose of 1.5 g).
  - – Indicated in patients with prior liver disease, diabetes, obesity, alcoholics, and intravenous drug users and in patients with hepatitis B and C infection.
    - ▪ Indicated above a cumulative dose of 1.5 g
  - – If liver biopsy indicates **(Table 12.1)**:
    - ▪ Up to grade IIIA liver changes, Mtx can be continued, but in such patients a liver biopsy should be repeated after every additional 1 g of Mtx or 6 months of continuous therapy.
    - ▪ In Grade IIIB and IV liver changes, further Mtx should not be given; however in exceptional cases with these changes, it may be continued with careful follow-up of liver biopsies.
- ○ Noninvasive methods: To detect early fibrosis or precirrhotic changes are:
  - – Serum aminoterminal type III procollagen (PIIIP) estimation:[8]
    - ▪ Serial estimation of PIIIP at three monthly intervals may dispense off with the need of liver biopsy in 70% of patients. If levels of PIIIP are normal, then liver biopsy is not warranted. If levels are elevated, then a liver biopsy is done.

TABLE 12.1: Histopathological changes in liver.	
Grade I	Normal or mild fatty infiltration with portal inflammation and nuclear variability
Grade II	Moderate-to-severe fatty infiltration with portal inflammation and widening, nuclear variability and necrosis
Grade III:	
A:	Mild fibrosis of liver
B:	Moderate-to-severe fibrosis
Grade IV	Cirrhosis of liver

---

[8]*Serum aminoterminal type III procollagen (PIIIP) estimation*: Unreliable in the presence of arthritis.

- Increased level of PIIIP indicates liver fibrosis, but it is a poor predictor for development of cirrhosis.
- However, like routine LFTs, PIIIP is not absolutely sensitive for identifying significant liver damage.
  - Magnetic resonance imaging (MRI) is of no value as a screening procedure for detecting Mtx-induced liver toxicity.

Instructions to Patients

Contraception

- Male patients are advised to use contraception to avoid pregnancy in partners for 3 months after stopping Mtx, because it causes abnormalities of sperms (mutagenic).
- Female patients are advised to use contraception to prevent pregnancy for one ovulatory cycle after stopping Mtx, because it is teratogenic and mutagenic.
- Patients advised to take 5 mg of folic acid, weekly to reduce nausea and vomiting and also to reduce hematological side effects (anemia).
- Patients advised to avoid concomitantly taking certain drugs,[9] which increase toxicity/side effects of Mtx.
- Patients should avoid consuming alcohol.

Response

The response to Mtx depends on the type of psoriasis being treated:

- *Chronic plaque psoriasis*: Though response is satisfactory, the improvement is slow and becomes obvious only after 3–4 weeks.
- *Erythroderma*: Though the response is not dramatic, the patient begins to feel better in about 7–10 days.
- *Generalized pustular psoriasis*: Response is dramatic as the constitutional symptoms including fever respond and pustules disappear within 48 hours. However, a new crop (though less severe) of pustules may appear in about 6–7 days.
- *Psoriatic arthropathy*: Response is seen in 4–6 weeks.

---

[9]*Drugs to be avoided*: Salicylates (aspirin), sulfonamides, tetracyclines, phenytoin, barbiturates, diuretics (frusemide), probenecid, and corticosteroids and other immunosuppressives.

Preparations Available

- *Tablets*: Mtx is available as tablets (2.5 mg, 5 mg, 7.5 mg, and 10 mg). Also available in combination with folic acid.
- *Injection*: 5–100 mg/mL

New Developments

Piritrexim

- A new dihydrofolate reductase inhibitor has been tried for the treatment of psoriasis.
- It causes only minimal side effects, since it is not stored inside the cell.
- Dose of 25–100 mg, twice daily for 5 days in a week. Repeated after 1 week.
- Response is satisfactory and side effects like nausea, malaise, and chills are minimal.

Topical Methotrexate

- Earlier studies failed to show response of psoriasis to topical Mtx.
- Newer modes of delivery include:
  - Using penetration enhancers such as decyl methyl sulfoxide, laurocapram, propylene glycol, and isopropyl alcohol.
  - Use of microemulsion is even better than delivery from aqueous solution.
- Use of 0.25% and 1% in hydrophilic gel has been found clinically effective and well-tolerated.

Cyclosporin A

Cyclosporin A is comparable to drugs like Mtx, retinoids, and systemic PUVA in treatment of psoriasis.

History

- Cyclosporin A, an immunosuppressive agent, was first used in renal transplant patients in 1978.
- Efficacy in psoriasis was initially noted fortuitously in 1979 and since then usefulness in psoriasis was established.

Mechanism of Action

Cyclosporin A acts in psoriasis by binding to cyclophilin, and this complex blocks calcineurin. This reduces the effect of nuclear factor of activated T-cells, inhibiting IL-2 and other cytokines.

Pharmacokinetics

- *Absorption*: CsA is insoluble in water. With soft gelatin capsule, the absorption is erratic and bioavailability is approximately 30%. The new microemulsion formulation has better absorption and bioavailability and lower intrapatient and interpatient variation and so better and predictable clinical efficacy.
- *Bioavailability*: Peak blood level occurs 2–4 hours after oral intake with average serum half-life of 18 hours. With microemulsion formulation, the peak serum level occurs 1 hour earlier than with the older formulation.
- *Excretion*: The drug is metabolized by the cytochrome P450 system in liver with an enterohepatic circulation. Metabolites of drug are inactive and 6% of drug is excreted in urine.
- *Drug interactions*: Concomitant administration of several drugs alters (increases or decreases) the efficacy and may increase the toxicity of CsA:
  - Drugs which increase blood levels of CsA: By inhibition of cytochrome P450 enzyme system. These drugs increase toxicity of CsA, e.g., erythromycin, azole group of antifungals (ketoconazole, fluconazole, and itraconazole), danazol, calcium channel blockers (verapamil, diltiazem), cimetidine, steroid hormones, and diuretics (furosemide and thiazides).
  - Drugs which decrease blood level of CsA: By inducing cytochrome p450 enzyme system to decrease efficacy of CsA, e.g., anticonvulsants (carbamazepine, phenytoin, and barbiturates), antibiotics (norfloxacin, acyclovir, and doxycycline), and phenylbutazone.
  - Drugs which alter renal function: For example, aminoglycosides, sulfonamides, diuretics, nonsteroidal anti-inflammatory drugs (NSAIDs), amphotericin B, and melphalan.

Side Effects and Management

Use of CsA is frequently associated with side effects.

Nephrotoxicity

- Manifests as elevation of serum creatinine.
- Develops in 25% of patients.
- Two types of CsA-induced nephrotoxicity seen:
  - *Reversible:* Which begins 2–3 weeks after drug initiation, associated with increased levels of serum creatinine and hypertension, and there is complete recovery on dose lowering or discontinuation of CsA.
  - *Irreversible:* A cumulative subclinical chronic toxicity usually manifests later and may occur in the absence of detectable elevation of serum creatinine or hypertension.
  - Calcium channel antagonists beneficial in CsA-induced hypertension and nephrotoxicity.

Hypertension

- Dose-dependent hypertension develops usually after 2 months of therapy.
- It is treated successfully with calcium channel blockers (nifedipine and nicardipine), which may actually prevent CsA-induced nephrotoxicity. However, some calcium channel blockers like verapamil and diltiazem are best avoided as they increase levels of CsA. Also important to avoid potassium-sparing diuretics due to risk of hyperkalemia.

Neurological Effects

- Like paresthesia and tremors are not uncommon and occur within 2 months of therapy.
- Headache, usually self-limiting, is frequent in patients with history of migraine.

Infections

Patients receiving CsA are at an increased risk of acquiring localized and generalized infections (viral, bacterial, fungal, and parasitic). Preexisting infections may get aggravated and fatal outcomes are reported.

Risk of Malignancy

Though there are reports of skin cancers, this is uncommon and probably related to previous ultraviolet radiation (UVR) exposure in patients with psoriasis.

Mucocutaneous Side Effects

- *Hypertrichosis*: It occurs in almost all, not limited to androgen sensitive areas and does not reverse with withdrawal.
- *Gingival hyperplasia*: It is seen in 70% of patients. More common in children, those with poor oral hygiene and those receiving concomitant calcium channel drugs. It responds to topical/ systemic azithromycin and metronidazole.
- *Acneiform eruption*: It can occur anytime, but more frequent in the first month of treatment. Monomorphic (comedonal or cystic) lesions.

Miscellaneous Side Effects

Nausea, diarrhea, anorexia, hyper-/hypokalemia, and hyperlipidemia have been reported.

Use in Pregnancy/Lactation/Children

- Pregnancy category C
- Probably safe in lactation
- Higher dose (5–7 mg/kg daily) used in children due to increased renal clearance

Use in Psoriasis

Indications

Cyclosporin A is indicated, when drugs like Mtx, PUVA, and acitretin cannot be used in patients with:
- Generalized pustular psoriasis
- Erythrodermic psoriasis
- Recalcitrant and extensive psoriasis
- Highly inflamed and eczematous type of psoriasis
- Severe psoriatic arthritis (though, it is only moderately effective)

Contraindications

Cyclosporin A is *contraindicated* in patients:
- With severe hypertension
- With renal disease and abnormal renal function tests
- Who are immunosuppressed, e.g., patients with psoriasis who have an underlying HIV infection
- With hypersensitivity to CsA
- With a cured or present malignancy
- Who have an active infection (relative contraindication)

Treatment Protocols

Dose

- Dose of CsA varies from 2 to 5 mg/kg/day (usually $\simeq$4 mg/kg/day). For calculating the dose, it is the *ideal body weight* and not the actual body weight which is used.
- The initial dose also depends on area of involvement and type of lesions:
  - *Erythrodermic and pustular psoriasis:* Higher dose is recommended for prompt relief of symptoms.
  - *Chronic plaque psoriasis*: Lower dose is recommended.

Dose Schedule

Two treatment schedules are available:
- *Low to high regimen is*:
  - Start with lower dose of 2.5 mg/kg/day
  - Gradually increase dose, by 0.5–1 mg/kg/day every 2 weeks up to a maximum of 4–5 mg/kg/day
  - Tapering recommended on improvement at 4 weekly intervals
- *High to low regimen is*:
  - Start with higher dose of 4–5 mg/kg/day, till adequate control is achieved.
  - Gradually decrease dose by 0.5–1 mg/kg/day every 2 weeks, to the lowest effective dose or treatment with CsA is stopped.

Monitoring Patients on Cyclosporin A (Flowchart 12.2)

Pretreatment Evaluation

- Assess the severity of psoriasis.
- *Blood pressure*: At least two normal baseline readings.

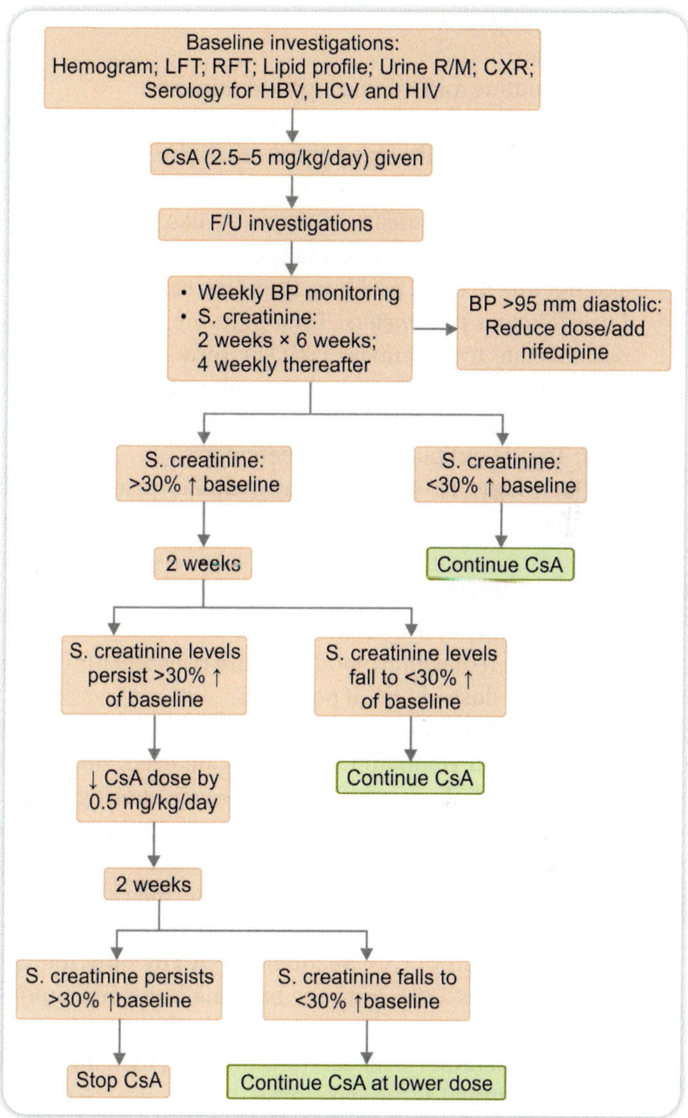

Flowchart 12.2: Algorithm for monitoring patients on cyclosporin A (CsA).

(CXR: chest X-ray; F/U: follow-up; HBV: hepatitis B virus; HCV: hepatitis C virus; HIV: human immunodeficiency virus; LFT: liver function test; RFT: renal function test; R/M: routine/microscopy)

- *Baseline investigations*:
    - Hemogram
    - *Urine:* Routine and microscopic examination
    - *Renal function parameters:* Serum creatinine,[10] blood urea and uric acid, with serum creatinine being the most important. Best to get two values of serum creatinine at baseline and use mean of the 2 as baseline level. If the baseline serum creatinine is raised because of erythroderma and not due to renal problem, then CsA can be given.
    - *Liver function parameters:* Total bilirubin, serum glutamate oxaloacetate transaminase (SGOT), serum glutamic pyruvic transaminase (SGPT), and alkaline phosphatase.
    - *Serum lipid profile:* Cholesterol and triglycerides.
    - *CXR:* To rule out pulmonary tuberculosis.
    - *HIV serology:* In high-risk individuals, prior to starting therapy.

Follow-up Evaluation

- Assess the severity of psoriasis.
- *Blood pressure:* If diastolic blood pressure rises >95 mm Hg then:
    - Reduce the dose of CsA, if possible.
    - Or add a calcium channel antagonist like nifedipine. Diltiazem and verapamil should not be used, because they inhibit metabolism of CsA. Potassium-sparing diuretics should also not be used for risk of developing hyperkalemia.
- *Investigations*: At follow-up visits include:
    - Renal function tests: Serum creatinine measurements are done every 2 weeks for 6 weeks and then every 4 weeks for the duration of CsA treatment. If at any time the serum creatinine rises >30% from the baseline,[11] it is repeated after 2 weeks.
    - If serum creatinine level falls to <30% more than the baseline, CsA is continued at the same dose.
    - If serum creatinine level persists at >30% from the baseline, the dose of CsA is reduced by 0.5 mg/kg/day and serum creatinine levels measured after 2 weeks.

---

[10]*Serum creatinine*: Earlier glomerular filtration rate was used.
[11]Even if it is within the normal range.

- If serum creatinine level continues to persist at >30% from the baseline, CsA is stopped.
- If serum creatinine level falls to <30% more than the baseline, CsA is continued at the lowered dose.

Response to Treatment

- In most patients, response is observed at 2–4 weeks, sometimes within the first 2 weeks.
- In most patients, PASI is reduced by 85% by 16 weeks.
- Withdrawal of therapy is frequently associated with relapse, but there is no rebound phenomenon.
- As CsA cannot usually be administered continuously for long periods at therapeutic doses (because of cost and toxicity), after controlling the acute phase with CsA, many physicians maintain the patient on PUVA or UVB. Though it is generally recommended that CsA and phototherapy should not be used simultaneously because of increased risk of skin malignancies, in actual practice there is need for an overlap period of about 2–3 weeks.

Advantages of Cyclosporin A

- Unlike Mtx, CsA is neither myelosuppressive nor potentially hepatotoxic and can be used in patients who have myelosuppression or hepatotoxicity.
- Unlike retinoids, CsA is not teratogenic (pregnancy category C). However, its routine use in pregnancy is best avoided.

Preparations Available

- *Capsules*: 25 mg, 50 mg, and 100 mg
- *Solutions*: 100 mg/mL
- *Injections*: 100 mg/mL

Retinoids

Retinoids are one of the safest long-term systemic therapies for psoriasis, despite plethora of side effects.

History

- Natural retinoids, e.g., vitamin A, were used in psoriasis with minimal improvement unless given in toxic doses.
- With arrival of oral retinoids, a new and potent approach to the treatment of psoriasis has become available.
- Oral retinoids used effectively in psoriasis include:
  - Etretinate (no longer available)
  - Acitretin
  - Isotretinoin[12]
  - Tazarotene

Mode of Action

In psoriasis, retinoids act through retinoic acid receptors (RARs)[13] by:

- Controlling growth and terminal differentiation of keratinocytes by regulating gene transcription.
- Reducing inflammation, partly through modification of arachidonic acid cascade.
- Modifying humoral and cellular responses, e.g., on polymorphonuclear cells.

Pharmacokinetics

- *Absorption*: Retinoids are absorbed like other fat-soluble molecules through formation of chylomicrons. Absorption is increased in presence of food.
- *Circulation*: Circulates bound to albumin.
- *Metabolism*: Retinoids are metabolized *via* oxidation to water-soluble products in the liver and excess is stored in the liver.
- *Specifically*:
  - Etretinate: It persists in body tissues, because it is lipophilic and poses a long-lasting risk of teratogenicity in women of child-bearing potential and hence has been withdrawn from the market.

---

[12]*Isotretinoin*: Most data on use of retinoids in psoriasis is on acitretin. There is no study comparing efficacy of acitretin vs. isotretinoin. The definite indication for use of isotretinoin in psoriasis is when it needs to be used in women of reproductive age group, because they can conceive 1 month after stopping isotretinoin but only 3 years after stopping acitretin.

[13]*RAR*: One of the two types of retinoid receptors, the other being retinoid X receptor (RXR).

- ○ Acitretin:
  - – Active metabolite of etretinate
  - – Has a short elimination half-life ($\simeq$50 hours) and so has lower potential for side effects. However, it is reverse esterified into etretinate in vivo, especially in the presence of alcohol, thereby substantially increasing its half-life.
  - – Therapeutic efficacy is similar to etretinate, but the dose of the latter needs to be lowered by approximately 20–33% for appropriate acitretin dosing.
- ○ *Tazarotene* is rapidly hydrolyzed to an inactive metabolite.
- *Drug interactions:* To reduce side effects and retain efficiency, it is important to avoid the following drug:
  - ○ Alcohol: It increases reverse esterification of acitretin into etretinate, warranting prolonged contraception.
  - ○ Vitamin A: It potentiates RAR-activity (leading to hyper-vitaminosis A). If at all needed, no more than 5,000 IU of vitamin A should be consumed per day concomitantly.
  - ○ Methotrexate: Due to hepatotoxicity.
  - ○ Tetracyclines: To avoid risk of pseudotumor cerebri and photosensitivity.
  - ○ Antidiabetics: Because retinoids may trigger hypoglycemia in patients on glibenclamide.
  - ○ Progestin mini pill: It has reduced efficiency in presence of retinoids and so should not be used for contraception in patients on retinoids.
  - ○ Drugs which inhibit cytochrome P450 enzyme system: Increase retinoid toxicity, e.g., macrolides[14] (erythromycin and clarithromycin) and azole group of antifungals (ketoconazole, fluconazole, and itraconazole).
  - ○ Drugs which induce cytochrome P450 enzyme system: Decrease efficacy of retinoids, e.g., anticonvulsants (carbamazepine, phenytoin, and barbiturates), antibiotics (norfloxacin, acyclovir, doxycycline), and phenylbutazone.
  - ○ Drugs which compete with P450 enzyme system: CsA levels may increase in patients taking retinoids.

---

[14]*Macrolides*: Of the macrolides, azithromycin does not inhibit P450 system.

Side Effects and Management

Acitretin is a patient-friendly drug with an extremely favorable risk–benefit ratio. However, clinical use of retinoids should be carefully monitored.

Teratogenicity

- Acitretin is highly teratogenic[15] (pregnancy category X) and women in reproductive age group should not generally be prescribed. If at all used in women of the reproductive age, isotretinoin is the preferred retinoid, and it too is absolutely contraindicated in:
  - Pregnant women
  - Lactating women
  - In women unwilling to comply with two methods of contraception
- In women, a prescription for retinoids *should not be given unless* the patient meets *all* the following conditions:
  - *Negative pregnancy test:* Two negative urine/serum pregnancy tests with a sensitivity of at least 25 mIU/mL:
    - First (screening) test, done when the decision to start acitretin is made.
    - Second (confirmation) test should be done depending on the patient's menstrual cycle.
      - In menorrheic patients, within 5 days of the menstrual period immediately preceding the initiation of acitretin.
      - In amenorrheic patients, done at least 11 days after the last act of unprotected sexual intercourse (i.e., intercourse without using two effective forms of contraception simultaneously).
  - Patient has agreed to use two effective methods of contraception (of which at least one is primary form)[16] simultaneously, unless abstinence is the chosen method or the

---

[15] *Teratogenic*: Causes retinoid embryopathy.

[16] *Primary forms of contraception*: Tubal ligation, partner's vasectomy, intrauterine devices, birth control pills, and injectable/implantable/insertable birth control products. Secondary forms of contraception: Latex condoms (± spermicide), diaphragms, and cervical caps (+ spermicide).

patient has had hysterectomy or is clearly postmenopausal. Patients who have undergone tubal ligation should also use a second method of contraception. Contraception should be started 1 month before starting treatment and continued throughout the duration of treatment and for at least 3 years[17] after acitretin has been stopped.

- Pregnancy testing and contraception counseling should be repeated at 4–weekly intervals while on therapy and 12 weekly for 3 years after treatment has been stopped.
- Women patients are advised to avoid alcohol while on treatment and for 2 months following discontinuation of therapy.

Mucocutaneous Side Effects

- Seen in almost all patients, being a sensitive indicator of patient compliance.
- Include:
  - *Cheilitis, gingivitis, and stomatitis*: Due to activation of RAR receptors
  - Photosensitivity
  - *Retinoid dermatitis:* Peeling of skin of palms and soles, dry skin, and pruritus.
  - *Hair loss:* Due to shortening of anagen phase leading to an increased telogen count as well as due to delay in onset of anagen phase.
- Are dose related, occurring more frequently with higher doses.
- Are usually acceptable to the patients because of the excellent response of psoriasis to retinoids. Also diminish with continued use and usually do not warrant discontinuation of drug.
- *Treatment*:
  - Cheilitis: With the use of lip balms containing sunscreens
  - Photosensitivity: With use of sunscreens
  - Dryness and pruritus: With use of emollients
  - Vitamin E coadministration probably has no protective effect against mucocutaneous side effects.[18]

---

[17] *For isotretinoin*: One month after isotretinoin is stopped. The pregnancy prevention program with acitretin goes with name of Do Your P.A.R.T while that with isotretinoin goes with the FDA mandated, iPLEDGE program.

[18] *Vitamin E*: Though earlier routinely used, recent studies have doubted efficacy of vitamin E in reducing mucocutaneous side effects.

Ophthalmic Side Effects

- Seen in 25% of patients.
- Dryness of eyes, which manifests as redness, burning and watering of eyes.
- Decreased night vision, and so patients should be warned about driving at night.
- Patients are advised not to use contact lenses during the course of treatment.
- *Ophthalmic side effects reduced by:* Using saline drops or artificial tears.

Hepatotoxicity[19]

- Transaminitis is seen in 25% of patients, but biopsy-proven toxic hepatitis is very rare.
- Patients with diabetes, obesity, and those consuming alcohol are at an increased risk of hepatotoxicity. Patients on acitretin are advised to avoid alcohol intake during treatment and for 2 months thereafter.
- In most patients, elevation of transaminases is mild-to-moderate and returns to normal even on continuation of therapy.
- If transaminases are elevated more than thrice the normal, acitretin should be stopped.

Serum Lipids

- Rise in serum lipids (most frequently in triglyceride fraction) is seen in 25% of patients. The rise stabilizes at 6–8 weeks.
- Risk factors for developing hypertriglyceridemia include obesity, diabetes mellitus, family history of hyperlipidemia, and alcohol intake.
- If the triglyceride fraction (more frequently) or cholesterol (less frequently) is elevated, then it is managed as follows:
    - *If mild elevation:* Taking a low fat and carbohydrate diet.
    - *If moderate elevation:* Using lipid lowering agents.
    - *If severe elevation:* Withdrawing acitretin.

---

[19]*Hepatotoxicity:* Usually an idiosyncratic drug-induced hepatitis. Recently cholestatic hepatitis reported.

Musculoskeletal System

- Not frequent
- Manifests as arthralgia, muscle pain (more in people undertaking strenuous work), ligamentous calcification, bone demineralization, premature closure of epiphyses, and osteophyte formation and rarely as diffuse idiopathic skeletal hyperostosis (DISH) if used for long periods of time.
- Patients who are likely to take acitretin for a long period should be monitored with a baseline X-ray of spine,[20] which should be repeated if patient develops symptoms.[21]

Neurological Side Effects

- Associated with features of pseudotumor cerebri (benign intracranial hypertension)
- Increased risk with concomitant use of tetracyclines, so avoid
- Manifests as headache, nausea, and vomiting
- If papilledema is noticed on ophthalmologic examination, then acitretin should be discontinued.

Pregnancy/Lactation/Children

- Avoid in lactation
- Has extensively been used in ichthyosiform dermatoses in children

Use in Psoriasis

Indications

Acitretin is a patient-friendly drug and carries an extremely favorable risk–benefit ratio and is indicated in the following:
- *Pustular psoriasis*:
  - Used in patients with pustular psoriasis in whom Mtx is contraindicated.
  - Response is rapid.

---

[20]*X-ray spine*: Some physicians prefer an ankle film. But there are no guidelines regarding baseline and annual radiographic monitoring during long-term oral retinoid therapy.

[21]*Repeat X-ray*: Some recommend 6-monthly X-rays.

- *Erythrodermic psoriasis*:
  - ○ Used in patients with erythrodermic psoriasis in whom Mtx is contraindicated.
  - ○ Response is slower than in pustular psoriasis.
- *Palmoplantar pustulosis*: Effective, although a few patients relapse soon after stopping treatment.
- *Extensive plaque psoriasis*: Which has responded inadequately to PUVA or UVB. Though plaque and guttate psoriasis are less responsive, retinoids can dramatically improve the response of these forms of psoriasis to PUVA and UVB. Also effective in maintenance of remission.
- *HIV-positive patients with extensive psoriasis:* Acitretin is the drug of choice, because it is not an immunosuppressive but an immunomodulator.
- *Psoriatic arthritis:* Conflicting reports on the efficacy of retinoids in the treatment of psoriatic arthritis.

Contraindications

Acitretin is *absolutely contraindicated* in:
- In pregnant and lactating women.
- In women in reproductive age, not willing to comply with two methods of contraception.

Acitretin is *preferably avoided* in:
- Patients with severe liver or renal impairment.
- In patients who are obese, have diabetes, or are not willing to give up alcohol during course of treatment.
- In males who are planning to father a child, even though it does not alter the sperms.

Treatment Protocols

Retinoids can be used as monotherapy as well as combination therapy.

Monotherapy

- *Initiating dose*: Standard dose is 0.25–0.6 mg/kg/day, up to a maximum of 1 mg/kg/day (25–50 mg/day). Higher doses are needed in pustular psoriasis, erythrodermic psoriasis, and recalcitrant hyperkeratotic palmoplantar psoriasis. Milk and food enhance absorption of acitretin.

- *Maintenance dose*: After control, patients can be maintained on 0.1–0.4 mg/kg/day.

Combination Therapy

The less than satisfactory response of some forms of psoriasis (e.g., extensive plaque psoriasis) to a retinoid alone has led to the use of combination therapies.

- *With phototherapy and photochemotherapy*:
  - RePUVA, is a combination of retinoids and PUVA and ReUVB, is a combination of retinoids and UVB.
  - Retinoids reduce epidermal thickness and so enhance the effects of phototherapy and photochemotherapy. Combination results in:
    - Clearance in patients who were earlier resistant to phototherapy and photochemotherapy.
    - Decrease in cumulative UV dose.
    - Reduced number and duration of treatments of PUVA.
    - Reduction of acitretin induced side effects.
    - Reduction of development of skin malignancies (by protection).
  - Dose for acitretin with phototherapy/photochemotherapy is 0.3 mg/kg/day.
  - Best results are obtained when the retinoids are administered about 2 weeks before initiating phototherapy/photochemotherapy.
- *With dithranol*: Plaques previously resistant to dithranol respond after addition of a retinoid.
- *With topical steroids*: Combination of oral retinoids with topical steroids is also effective.
- *With systemic agents:* A combination of acitretin (25 mg daily) and hydroxyurea (500 mg twice daily) has been found effective in chronic plaque psoriasis and pustular psoriasis.

Monitoring Patients on Retinoids (Flowchart 12.3)

Pretreatment Evaluation

- Assess the severity of psoriasis.
- Specifically ask for history of hypertension, diabetes, hyperlipidemias, cardiovascular, or neurovascular episodes.

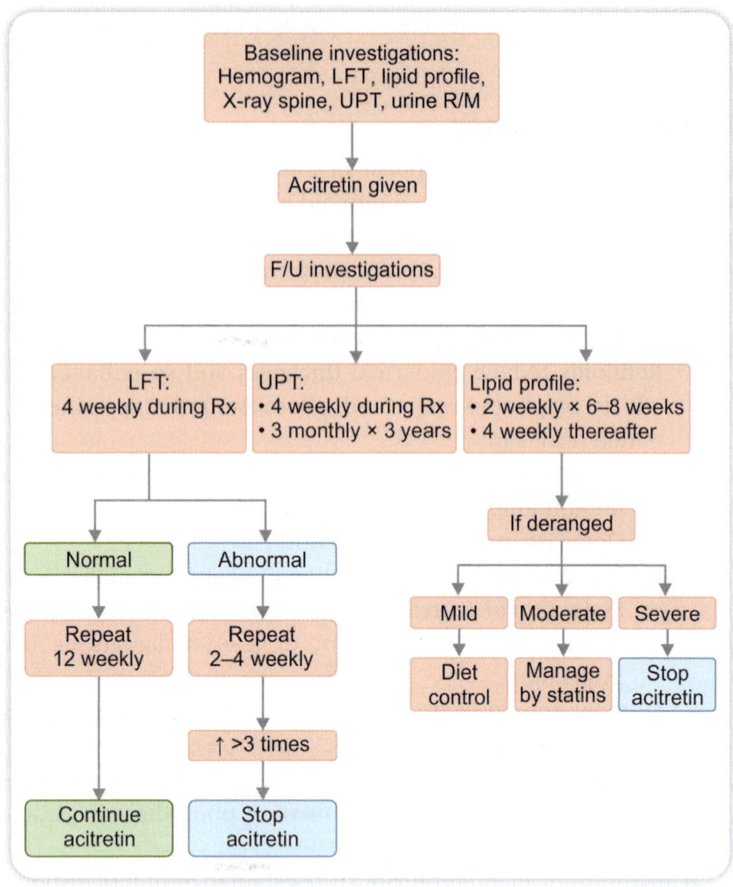

Flowchart 12.3: Algorithm for monitoring patients on acitretin.

(F/U: follow-up; LFT: liver function test; R/M: routine/microscopy; UPT: urine pregnancy test)

- In women patients, rule out pregnancy and lactation and enquire about menstrual cycle and use of contraception.
- *Baseline investigations include*:
  - Complete hemogram
  - LFTs
  - Renal function tests (urea, creatinine)
  - Lipid profile
  - Urine analysis

- X-ray of spine,[20,21] if it is planned to give acitretin for more than 6 months
- Pregnancy test in women in reproductive age group.

Follow-up Evaluations (At 4-weekly Intervals)

- Assess severity of psoriasis.
- In female patients of reproductive age, pregnancy ruled out at each visit by history and by a pregnancy test. Counsel patient on regular use of two effective methods of contraception at every visit.

Follow-up investigations include:

- *Urine pregnancy test:* Every 4 weeks while on treatment, then 12 weekly for 3 years.
- *LFTs:* It should first be repeated at 4 weeks and then:
  - If normal, repeat at 12 weekly intervals.
  - If abnormal, repeat at 2–4 weekly intervals, depending on degree of transaminitis.
  - Stop acitretin, if transaminases are elevated more than *thrice* normal.
- *Lipid profile*: It should be repeated at:
  - 2-weekly intervals, until the lipid levels stabilize (usually in 6–8 weeks).
  - After lipid levels have stabilized, repeat at 4 weekly intervals.
- *Radiographic evaluation*: It is important to carefully enquire for possible skeletal pain and mobility restrictions. If the patient is symptomatic, then a repeat X-ray of spine needs to be done.

Response

Depends on the type of psoriasis:

- *Pustular psoriasis:* Responds in 1–2 weeks.
- *Erythrodermic psoriasis*: Responds in 3–4 weeks.
- *Chronic plaque psoriasis:* Improvement occurs gradually, requiring up to 3–6 months for complete response. There may even be an initial flare, lasting 3–6 weeks.

Preparations Available

Available as capsules 10 mg and 25 mg.

Hydroxyurea

History

- Hydroxyurea is an antimetabolite agent used in treatment of myeloma and myelogenous leukemia.
- It was introduced as a second-line treatment modality in psoriasis in 1965.

Mode of Action

- Primary mechanism of action is unknown.
- It is an antimetabolite agent, which inhibits synthesis of DNA without significantly inhibiting RNA and protein synthesis.

Pharmacokinetics

- Readily absorbed after oral administration. Effect of food on absorption not known.
- Reaches peak concentration by 2 hours. Rapidly excreted by kidney within 24 hours.

Use in Psoriasis

Indications

- Second-line therapy for treatment of extensive psoriasis (>20% BSA involved) in whom Mtx, cyclosporin, and acitretin are contraindicated.
- Ineffective in pustular and erythrodermic psoriasis.

Contraindications

- Pregnant and lactating mothers
- Women of childbearing age, who have not completed their family, because of its mutagenic potential.
- Children, because safety in pediatric age is not established.

Treatment Protocol

Dose

- Initial adult dose of 0.5 g daily, as single or in divided doses
- Weekly increment of 0.5 g, if no response at 2 weeks, up to a maximum of 2 g daily

Monitoring Patient on Hydroxyurea (Flowchart 12.4)

Pretreatment Assessment

- Assess the severity of psoriasis.
- In female patients, rule out pregnancy (category D drug) and lactation.
- *Baseline investigations include*:
  - Hemogram (total leukocyte and platelet counts)
  - Renal function tests (blood urea and serum creatinine)
  - LFTs
  - Lipid profile
  - Urine analysis
  - HIV status

Follow-up Evaluation

- Assess the severity of psoriasis **(Flowchart 12.4)**.
- Follow-up investigations include:

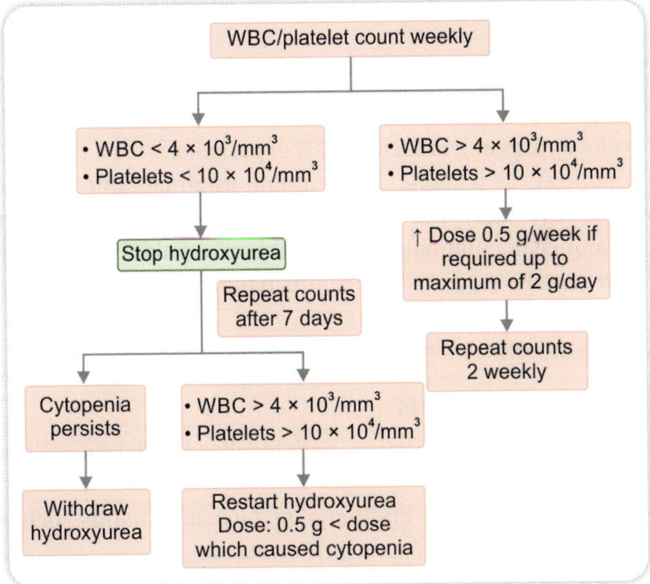

Flowchart 12.4: Algorithm for monitoring patients on hydroxyurea.
(WBC: white blood cell)

- o Hemogram repeated after 1 week:
  - – If total leukocyte count is >4,000/mm^3 and platelet count >100,000/mm^3, the dose of hydroxyurea is increased (if required) and counts repeated at weekly intervals.
  - – When the maximum/therapeutically optimum dose (2 g) is reached and the cell counts (leukocyte and platelet) remains normal, the counts are then repeated at 2-weekly intervals throughout the course of therapy.
  - – If at any time leukocyte count falls <4,000/mm^3 or platelet count falls <100,000/mm^3, hydroxyurea is stopped and the counts repeated after 7 days.
  - – If the cell counts return to normal, hydroxyurea is restarted at 0.5 g lower than the dose which caused cytopenia.
  - – If the cytopenia persists, hydroxyurea is withdrawn.

Response

- Improvement is slow, starting after a couple of weeks.
- If after 2 weeks there is no improvement, daily dose increased weekly by 0.5 g up to a maximum 2 g.

Adverse Effects

Myelosuppression

- Myelosuppression is seen in 10% of patients.
- It manifests as leukopenia (frequent, minimal almost universal which invariably precedes thrombocytopenia and anemia), megaloblastic anemia, or thrombocytopenia (less frequent). Bone marrow suppression is more in patients previously exposed to radiation and chemotherapy.
- It is rapidly reversible on reducing dose.

Cutaneous Side Effects

- *Pigmentation*: Pigmentation, both localized and diffused, is seen in 6% of patients.
- Rarely nail changes, erythema of face and hands, lichenoid eruption, and actinic psoriasis may occur.

Miscellaneous Effects

- Potentially teratogenic drug which is best avoided in women of child bearing age.

- Decreased fertility with long-term therapy has been reported.
- Safety and effectiveness in pediatric patients is not established.

Preparations Available

Hydroxyurea is available as capsules 0.25 and 0.5 g.

Systemic Corticosteroids

Systemic corticosteroids are not routinely recommended in the treatment of psoriasis because of rebound on withdrawal. However, these may be needed to be given in certain circumstances.

Adverse Effects

Cutaneous Adverse Effects

- Acneiform eruption
- Striae
- Hirsutism
- Rebound on withdrawal, even pustular lesions

Systemic Adverse Effects

- Increased susceptibility to infection
- Hypertension
- Diabetes
- Obesity
- Cataract

Use in Psoriasis

- *Impetigo herpetiformis*: This is a definite indication for the use of systemic steroids, given either alone or in combination with dapsone. Given in a dose of 1 mg/kg prednisolone equivalent with gradual tapering of dose as patient responds. The response is dramatic and fetal wastage is reduced.
- *Generalized pustular psoriasis*: When patient is toxic, very sick, Mtx, acitretin, and cyclosporin cannot be used.
- *Mutilating psoriatic arthropathy*: Corticosteroids have been shown to provide symptomatic relief in psoriatic arthropathy, but it has been observed that on withdrawal, the patient may have severe rebound phenomenon. So, the use of oral steroids is

limited to patients with mutilating psoriatic arthropathy. In these patients, steroids can be given as:
- *Daily dose*: Initially with prednisolone 30–40 mg daily tapered over 4–8 weeks.
- *Weekly pulse therapy:* As oral mini pulse of betamethasone 5 mg, 1–2 doses/week.
- *Monthly pulse therapy:* Of oral betamethasone, 100 mg or intravenous dexamethasone, 100 mg daily for 3 consecutive days every month.

Fumaric Acid Esters

History

Fumarates have been in use in Northern Europe for 30 years for the treatment of moderately severe psoriasis.

Pharmacokinetics

- Absorption is more consistent and better when taken 1 hour before food.
- After absorption, drug hydrolyzed to monomethyl fumarate, the main active metabolite.

Mode of Action

Fumaric acid esters act in psoriasis by:
- Switching Th1 dominated response to Th2 response.
- Inhibiting keratinocyte proliferation.

Use in Psoriasis

Indications

- Severe psoriasis with >25% BSA involvement
- Frequent relapses
- Psoriasis resistant to conventional therapy
- Severe psoriatic arthritis
- *Nail psoriasis:* Though nail psoriasis responds to fumarate esters, the drug *should not be used only to treat nail psoriasis.*

Contraindications

- Patients with severe gastrointestinal disease and hepatic dysfunction
- Patients with renal impairment
- Patients with malignancies and hematological impairment
- Patients <18 years of age
- Pregnant and lactating mothers

Adverse Effects

Gastrointestinal Side Effects

- Gastrointestinal side effects are common (>50% of patients).
- The side effects include nausea, diarrhea, and tenesmus.
- Side effects are reduced by administering domperidone, half an hour before fumarate esters.

Flushing

- Flushing is seen in a third of patients.
- It manifests as flushing, 1–6 hours after ingestion of drug.
- Self-limiting, becoming less prominent over course of treatment.

Nephrotoxicity

- Nephrotoxicity is seen infrequently.
- It results in tubular impairment and manifests as proteinuria and increased serum creatinine.
- It is reduced by drinking at least 2 L of water every day.

Hematopoietic

Lymphopenia and eosinophilia.

Treatment Protocol

Dose

Treatment is started with lower dose, increased over period of weeks:
- Initial dose, 30 mg/day of dimethyl fumarate increased weekly by 30 mg up to a maximum of 720 mg (in three divided doses), depending on response and patient's ability to tolerate the medication.
- Treatment is given for a maximum of 6 months.

Monitoring

Baseline and follow-up (4–8 weeks):
- Hemogram
- Urine, routine, and sediment

Response to Treatment

- A good clinical response is seen in about 75% of patients by 4–6th week; in these patients, PASI reduces by 80% at the end of 16 weeks.
- The response is poor in 25% of patients, either because the drug has to be withdrawn or given only in suboptimal doses due to side effects, or the drug is ineffective.

Preparations Available

Fumaric acid esters commercially available contain two fumaric acid esters:
- Dimethyl fumarate
- Ethyl hydrogen fumarate of Ca, Mg, and Zn

Mycophenolate Mofetil

History

- Mycophenolate mofetil (MM) was first approved by FDA in 1995 to prevent acute rejection after renal transplantation.
- Efficacy in psoriasis is demonstrated way back in 1970s and has been successfully used for the treatment of recalcitrant psoriasis.

Pharmacokinetics

- Oral absorption is rapid and complete. Preferably taken on empty stomach.
- MM is rapidly hydrolyzed to active metabolite mycophenolic acid, both after oral and intravenous administration.
- The drug is metabolized in the liver and is excreted in urine.

Mode of Action

Mycophenolic acid interferes with the production of precursors for the synthesis of DNA and RNA.

Adverse Effects

- Reasonably well tolerated in patients with psoriasis with the more frequent side effects (in 20% of patients) being gastrointestinal (nausea, vomiting, and diarrhea). Minimized by reducing or dividing the dose.
- Uncomplicated viral infections such as herpes zoster and herpes simplex may also occur.
- Infrequently causes anemia.

Use in Psoriasis

Indications

- Moderate–severe psoriasis in whom conventional systemic drugs such as Mtx, acitretin, and cyclosporin are contraindicated due to underlying liver/renal dysfunction.
- Great promise in patients with psoriatic arthropathy.

Treatment Protocol

Dose

1–2 g/day

Combination Therapy

Mycophenolate mofetil has been used in combination with CsA to reduce its nephrotoxicity.

Modified Regimens

Recently topical MM 2% cream has been found to be effective in reducing erythema, induration, and scaling in plaque psoriasis.

Monitoring

Baseline

- Hemogram, including complete blood count
- LFTs
- Renal function tests

Follow-up

- Hemogram including complete blood count weekly for 4 weeks, fortnightly for 8 weeks, and monthly thereafter. If total leukocyte

count (TLC) is <4,000/mm^3 or platelets <150,000/mm^3, then discontinue.
- LFTs are repeated as above.

Response

At a dose of 2 g daily, psoriasis responds in 4–6 weeks.

Preparations Available

Mycophenolate mofetil is available as tablets 250 mg and 500 mg.

Phosphodiesterase Inhibitors: Apremilast

History

Apremilast is an oral phosphodiesterase-4 (PDE-4) inhibitor approved by the US FDA in 2014 and by the Drug Controller General of India in 2017 for the management of moderate-to-severe plaque psoriasis and psoriatic arthritis.

Pharmacokinetics

- The absolute bioavailability is around 73%.
- It is metabolized by both cytochrome P450 (CYP)-mediated (mainly CYP3A4) oxidation and non-CYP mediated hydrolysis.
- Excretion is mainly through renal route.

Mode of Action

Apremilast inhibits PDE-4 which leads to accumulation of intracellular cyclic adenosine monophosphate (cAMP). The inhibition of PDE-4 leads to reduction of proinflammatory cytokines like tumor necrosis factor (TNF) alpha and interleukin 23 (IL-23) and increase in levels of anti-inflammatory mediators like IL-10.

Adverse Effects

Adverse effects include diarrhea (15–20% patients), nausea, upper respiratory infection, headache, and weight loss. It can cause worsening of depression.

Use in Psoriasis

Indications

- Moderate-to-severe plaque psoriasis
- Psoriatic arthritis

Treatment Protocol

- Recommended dose of apremilast is 30 mg twice daily orally.
- The treatment is started with 10 mg morning dose with a daily increment of 10 mg till required dose of 30 mg bd is reached. This dose titration is done to minimize the gastrointestinal side effects.
- In patients with renal impairment, the recommended dose is 30 mg once daily.

Response

Apremilast usually takes 4–6 weeks to show efficacy.

Preparations Available

Apremilast is available as tablets 10 mg, 20 mg, and 30 mg.

Janus Kinase Inhibitors: Tofacitinib

History

- Tofacitinib is an oral first-generation Janus kinase (JAK) inhibitor, which was approved for use in psoriatic arthritis in 2017.
- Phase 3 trials have shown efficacy in moderate-to-severe plaque psoriasis.

Pharmacokinetics

- Tofacitinib is rapidly absorbed after oral administration with half-life of 3 hours.
- It is metabolized by the hepatic CYP system, mainly the CYP3A4 enzyme.
- Elimination occurs via both hepatic (70%) and renal routes (30%).

Mode of Action

- Tofacitinib inhibits JAK1 and JAK3 enzymes, blocking intracellular signal pathway mediated by JAK and signal transducer and activator of transcription (STAT) proteins, thereby inhibiting gene transcription of proinflammatory cytokines.
- IL-12 and IL-23 are JAK/STAT-dependent cytokines, which are the principal mediators of psoriasis. Their upstream blockade by tofacitinib indirectly decreases IL–17 levels.

Adverse Effects

- Increased risk of infections; new onset/reactivation of latent infections
- Diarrhea, fatigue, dizziness, and headache
- Increased risk of malignancies
- *Laboratory abnormalities*: Hematological, liver derangement with enzyme elevations, and dyslipidemia
- Impaired response to vaccination

Preparations Available

Tofacitinib is available as tablets 5 mg, 10 mg, and 11 mg [extended release (XR)].

Tyrosine Kinase Inhibitors

- Deucravacitinib is an oral tyrosine kinase 2 inhibitor used in the treatment of moderate-to-severe plaque psoriasis.
- Tyrosine kinase 2 is involved in the signaling of cytokines involved in the pathogenesis of psoriasis such as IL-23. Deucravacitinib is involved in the inhibition of this pathway.
- *Use in psoriasis*:
    - FDA recommended the use of this drug in patients with moderate-to-severe plaque psoriasis who are candidates for systemic therapy or phototherapy.
    - Recommended dose of deucravacitinib is 6 mg once daily orally.
- *Side effects*: Upper respiratory infection is the most common side effect. Other very rare side effects are pericarditis and cholecystitis.

Miscellaneous and Experimental Drugs

Tacrolimus

- Tacrolimus is a hydrophobic macrolide lactone.
- It is a potent immunosuppressive agent that inhibits T-cell activation.
- *Use in psoriasis*:
  - Systemic tacrolimus is moderately effective in psoriasis while topical is not.
  - Initial dose is 0.05 mg/kg/day, which can be increased to 0.1 mg/kg/day at 3 weeks and to 0.15 mg/kg/day at 6 weeks.
- *Side effects*:
  - Diarrhea, insomnia, and paresthesias are frequent.
  - Hypertension, nephrotoxicity, and immunosuppression are less frequent.

Mycobacterium Vaccae

General Information

- *Mycobacterium vaccae* is a nonpathogenic, fast-growing mycobacterium found in soil.
- Heat killed suspension of *M. vaccae* has been used as adjunct therapy for mycobacterial diseases, especially tuberculosis and leprosy.

Mode of Action

Exact mechanism of action of *M. vaccae* in psoriasis is not known:

- It may polarize the immunologic balance toward a Th1 response.
- Increased production of anti-inflammatory cytokines such as transforming growth factors and IL-10.
- It may be related to mitigated effects of TNF.

Indications

Mycobacterium vaccae holds promise in the treatment for moderate-to-severe disease as it is nontoxic and effective.

Treatment Protocol

Two doses of *M. vaccae* vaccine (containing approximately 5×10^8 heat killed organisms) given intradermally at 4 weekly intervals in the deltoid region induce remission in 50% of patients with moderate-to-severe psoriasis.

Liarozole

- Imidazole derivative
- It acts by inhibiting retinoic acid 4-hydroxylase activity, resulting in increased levels of endogenous all-trans retinoic acid.
- Effective in severe psoriasis at a dose of 150 mg twice daily.
- Side effects similar to those of retinoids.

Diphtheria Fusion Toxin (Denileukin Diftitox)

- It consists of IL-2 molecules attached to diphtheria toxin (DAB 389 IL–2).
- It binds to high affinity IL-2 receptors on activated T-cells, thereby destroying them.
- Side effects are severe.

Other Investigational Drugs

- Ponesimod is a sphingosine phosphate receptor-1 inhibitor that has shown to be effective in the treatment of plaque psoriasis in early clinical trials.
- Baricitinib is another analog of tofacitinib that has been found to be effective in psoriasis.
- Other investigational therapies useful in the treatment of psoriasis include exenatide (glucagon-like peptide 1 analog).

Biologicals Therapy

Introduction

Biologicals are large protein molecules that target very specific parts of the immune path and so (at least theoretically) have fewer side-effects than other immunosuppressive drugs. Biologicals are generally divided into three major groups based on their structure:
1. Monoclonal antibodies, e.g., infliximab, adalimumab
2. Fusion antibody protein, e.g., etanercept
3. Recombinant human cytokines and growth factor, e.g., oprelvekin

Principles of Use of Biologicals

Biologicals used in psoriasis target two selective areas of pathogenesis **(Table 13.1)**:
1. *T-cell activation inhibitors:* These drugs block the binding of antigen presenting cells to T-cells, (a process mediated by costimulatory molecules) thereby inhibiting T-cell activation, e.g., alefacept, efalizumab.
2. *Inflammatory cytokine inhibitors:* These drugs inhibit cytokines directly involved in the inflammation process associated with psoriasis. Tumor necrosis factor alpha (TNF-α) inhibitors such as adalimumab and infliximab target TNF-α to reduce inflammation, while interleukin (IL)-12/23 inhibitors such as ustekinumab and IL-17 inhibitors such as secukinumab address other specific cytokines critical in psoriasis.

TABLE 13.1: Mechanism of action of biologicals in psoriasis.

TNF-α inhibitors	Adalimumab, infliximab, etanercept, and golimumab
IL-12/23 inhibitors	Ustekinumab and briakinumab
IL-23 inhibitors	Tildrakizumab and guselkumab
IL-17 inhibitors	Secukinumab, ixekizumab, and brodalumab
Inhibition of IL-6	Tocilizumab
Inhibition of IL-1	Anakinra
Reduction of primary stimulation of T-cells	Teplizumab and otelixizumab[1]
Interrupting costimulatory signal	Alefacept[2] and efalizumab[3]
Targeting T-cell proliferation	Daclizumab and basiliximab[4]

(IL: interleukin; TNF-α: tumor necrosis factor alpha)

Indications for Biologicals

Treatment with biologicals for psoriasis is recommended[5] for patients with severe disease and meet at least one criterion from the clinical categories.

- *Severe psoriasis:* Patients must have severe psoriasis, which is typically indicated by:
  - A Psoriasis Area and Severity Index (PASI) score of ≥10, or
  - Body surface area (BSA) involvement of 10% or more, and
  - A Dermatology Life Quality Index (DLQI) score >10.

    Note: In certain cases, such as acral psoriasis affecting critical areas, patients may still be eligible even if these scores are lower.[6]
- *Additional clinical categories:* Patients should also meet at least one of the following conditions:

---

[1] Block CD3/CD4/CD8
[2] Anti-CD2, blocks APC LFA-3/CD2 interaction
[3] Monoclonal antibody against the CD11a subunit of LFA-1
[4] IL-2 inhibitors
[5] British Association of Dermatologists, 2009
[6] *Exceptional circumstances*: This includes cases where the disease severely affects high-impact sites, causing significant functional or psychological issues.

- ○ Cannot use or are at risk from standard therapies such as phototherapy[7] or systemic treatments[8] due to contraindications or potential severe side effects.
- ○ Intolerant to standard systemic therapy
- ○ Unresponsive to standard systemic therapy
- ○ Have other significant health conditions that make the use of certain systemic agents unsafe.
- ○ Have severe, unstable, or life-threatening disease.

Special Considerations for Skin and Joint Disease

- Active psoriatic arthritis or skin disease meeting British Society for Rheumatology (BSR) or British Association of Dermatologists (BAD) guideline criteria.
- Severe psoriasis and psoriatic arthritis, especially if methotrexate is unsuitable or ineffective, warranting consideration for biologicals due to the dual benefit.

Monitoring and Precautions

Although considered to be selective immunosuppressives, patients on biologicals need to be monitored for the development of infections and malignancies. And even though there are no standard guidelines, most dermatologists carry out a battery of "baseline" and "while on therapy" tests in patients with psoriasis who are being treated with biologicals:

- *Hemogram*: Including complete blood cell count and platelet count.
- *Liver function tests*: Including viral hepatitis panel.
- *Serious infection*: Ruling out active serious infections,[9] it being prudent to withhold the biologic until the infection has resolved. Screening for tuberculosis (TB) is mandatory especially with

---

[7] *Phototherapy limitations*: Inapplicable in cases such as exceeding safe exposure limits, non-responsiveness, rapid relapse, history of skin cancer or severe sunburn, intolerance to UV exposure (especially in sun-sensitive individuals), or logistical challenges.

[8] *Standard systemic therapy*: Includes drugs such as ciclosporin, methotrexate, and acitretin, with specific dosage guidelines.

[9] *Serious infection*: Defined as infection that requires antibiotic therapy.

TNF-α inhibitors at baseline and with variable frequencies thereafter.
- *Pregnancy category:* Efalizumab[10] is of pregnancy category C while alefacept, adalimumab, etanercept, and infliximab are all of pregnancy category B.
- *Vaccinations:* While on biologicals, patients are advised to avoid vaccination with live vaccines (varicella, mumps, measles, rubella, oral typhoid, and yellow fever) and live-attenuated vaccines (intranasal influenza and herpes zoster vaccine).

Tumor Necrosis Factor-alpha Inhibitors

The anti-TNF-α biologicals agents currently approved for the treatment of psoriasis and psoriatic arthritis (PsA) are etanercept, infliximab, adalimumab, and certolizumab.

Chemical Structure

- *Etanercept:* A fusion protein linking the TNF-α ligand binding domain to the (fragment, crystallizable) portion of human immunoglobulin G1 (IgG1).
- *Infliximab:* A chimeric monoclonal antibody combining a human IgG1 constant domain with a murine variable domain.
- *Adalimumab:* A fully human monoclonal antibody targeting TNF-α.

Mechanism of Action

These agents bind to TNF-α, blocking its interaction with receptors and inhibiting the inflammatory cascade that contributes to psoriasis pathology.

Pharmacokinetics

Infliximab has a half-life elimination between 7 and 12 days, adalimumab ranges from 10 to 20 days, etanercept is approximately 70–130 hours, and certolizumab possesses a half-life elimination around 14 days.

---

[10] *Efalizumab*: It has been withdrawn due to risk of progressive multifocal encephalopathy.

Indications

- Moderate-to-severe plaque psoriasis in adults
- Psoriatic arthritis

Contraindications

Absolute

History of allergic reaction to therapeutic agent or murine proteins.

Relative

- Untreated hepatitis B infection
- History of lymphoreticular malignancy
- Active infection (including TB) or sepsis
- Congestive heart failure (CHF) [New York Heart Association (NYHA) class III or IV]
- Preexisting or family history of demyelinating disease (including multiple sclerosis)

Available Formulations

- *Infliximab:* 100 mg lyophilized powder
- *Adalimumab:* 40 mg/0.8 mL prefilled syringe
- *Etanercept:* Available in two strengths, 25 mg/0.5 mL and 50 mg/mL prefilled syringes
- *Certolizumab:* 200 mg prefilled syringe

Dose and Administration (Table 13.2)

- Of all the TNF-α blockers, only infliximab is administered intra-venously while rest are given subcutaneously.
- *Infliximab*: Distributed in lyophilized concentrate; 100 mg in each 20-mL vial. It should be reconstituted with 10 mL of sterile water and dosed to 250 mL of 0.9% normal saline.

Adverse Events

Administration-related Reactions

- *Infusion reactions:* These occur in about 20% of patients receiving infliximab, often linked to antibody development.

TABLE 13.2: Dose and administration.

Biological agent	Loading dose	Maintenance
Infliximab	5 mg/kg IV infusion administered in week 0, week 2, and week 6	5 mg/kg IV infusion administered every 8 weeks
Adalimumab	80 mg subcutaneous injection (2 × 40 mg at the initial dose), followed by a 40 mg subcutaneous injection 1 week later	40 mg subcutaneous injection every 2 weeks
Etanercept	50 mg subcutaneous injection twice weekly for 12 weeks	50 mg subcutaneous injection once per week
Certolizumab	400 mg subcutaneous injection every 2 weeks	

- ○ Mild-to-moderate symptoms include fever, chills, pruritus, and urticaria. These can be managed by slowing or stopping the infusion, with possible administration of antihistamines, acetaminophen, or corticosteroids.
- ○ Severe reactions, though rare (1–3%), such as anaphylaxis (laryngeal edema, severe bronchospasm, and hypotension), necessitate discontinuation and immediate medical attention.
- *Injection site reactions:* Common with etanercept and adalimumab, typically in the first month and last for 3–5 days.
  - ○ Symptoms may include erythema, itching, pain, swelling, and hemorrhage.
  - ○ Managed with local cold packs, topical corticosteroids, and analgesia without needing to stop therapy.

Neutropenia

- Defined as neutrophils <2,000/mm^3.
- Neutropenia is usually seen after 2 weeks of therapy. The drop in neutrophil count is more with infliximab which may be because of bolus dose. Only 1% of patients with neutropenia develop serious infections.
- Therapy should be discontinued if the neutrophil count <500 mm^3.

Demyelinating Disease

- Tumor necrosis factor-alpha antagonists may cause neurological symptoms similar to demyelination and are contraindicated in patients with a personal or family history of demyelinating diseases.
- Possible symptoms include paresthesia, visual and gait disturbances, confusion, apraxia, facial palsy, and Guillain–Barré syndrome.
- Discontinue medication if these symptoms occur and conduct a thorough neurological evaluation, including:
  - Eye examination for optic neuritis
  - Magnetic resonance imaging (MRI) of the brain
  - Lumbar puncture for cerebrospinal fluid analysis, especially for oligoclonal bands and IgG levels.

Malignancies

- Anti-TNF agents are linked to a potential increase in lymphoma risk, highlighted by a Food and Drug Administration (FDA) black box warning.
- Subsequent research shows no significant increased lymphoma risk compared to disease-modifying antirheumatic drugs (DMARDs), though regular skin checks are advised due to a higher incidence of nonmelanoma skin cancers.

Congestive Heart Failure

- Tumor necrosis factor-alpha inhibitors may worsen outcomes in severe CHF, with initial studies suggesting higher mortality and hospitalization rates.
- They are not associated with an increased incidence of CHF onset but should be avoided in severe CHF patients.

Antidrug Antibodies/Biologic Fatigue

- Infliximab treatment may result in antidrug antibodies (ADAs) in up to 44% of patients within 6 months, while adalimumab shows a 19% incidence, rising to 28% over 3 years.
- Etanercept has a lower ADA incidence of 0–7%, with these antibodies typically being transient and non-neutralizing.

- Concurrent methotrexate use with infliximab can lower ADA development, and higher initial drug doses may also reduce ADA frequency.
- Patients developing ADAs may switch biologics to preserve treatment effectiveness.

Paradoxical Adverse Effects

- Paradoxical adverse effects (PAEs) emerge during biological treatment as either the exacerbation of conditions typically managed by these drugs (true PAEs) or the onset of certain immune-mediated conditions not yet proven to be treated by these drugs (borderline PAEs).
- True PAEs include worsening of psoriasis, inflammatory bowel disease (IBD), and hidradenitis suppurativa; borderline PAEs involve uveitis and vitiligo.
- Adalimumab may increase the risk of paradoxical psoriasis more than etanercept or infliximab.
- Management depends on severity:
  - Severe PAEs require stopping TNF-α therapy.
  - Mild cases may only need topical psoriasis treatments.
- Conditions covering >5% BSA or presenting as palmoplantar pustulosis may require changing TNF-α antagonists and using topical occlusive treatments.
- Uncontrolled PAEs might necessitate phototherapy or systemic treatments such as methotrexate.

Infections

- Tumor necrosis factor-alpha inhibitors increase infection risk in the first 6–12 months, especially with infliximab, and even more so in patients over 65 or on concurrent immunosuppressants.
- Infliximab may lead to earlier manifestation of mycobacterial infections such as TB compared to etanercept.
- Septic arthritis (*Staphylococcus aureus*) and listeriosis reports are higher with infliximab use.
- Adalimumab and infliximab are associated with a greater risk of *Legionella pneumonia.*
- Hepatitis B reactivation and higher herpes zoster infection risk linked to TNF-α inhibitors.

- Infliximab is associated with fungal infections such as histoplasmosis and coccidioidomycosis; the FDA recommends stopping the drug if such infections occur.

Mycobacterium Tuberculosis Infection

- Tumor necrosis factor-alpha inhibitors are associated with an increased risk of tuberculosis, ranging from 1.6 to 25.1 times higher than without these drugs, often presenting with extrapulmonary and disseminated TB.
- Mandatory pre-biologic TB screening includes prior TB history, clinical examination, chest X-ray, and tuberculin skin test (TST) or interferon gamma release assay (IGRA) tests.
- Treatment for latent TB infection is necessary if tests are positive, especially if past TB is indicated on a chest X-ray.
- Patients with latent TB require at least 1 month of anti-TB prophylaxis before biologics and regular monitoring thereafter.
- Active TB must be treated before commencing biologic therapy, completing the full anti-TB treatment regimen if possible.
- Latent tuberculosis; therapy recommendations and dose range **(Table 13.3)**

Human Immunodeficiency Virus

- Human immunodeficiency virus (HIV) patients without recent opportunistic infections can use TNF-α inhibitors if on effective highly active antiretroviral therapy (HAART) with normalized CD4 counts (>200 cells/cu.mm) and undetectable viral load.

TABLE 13.3: Recommendation of dose.

Drug	Dose/kg body weight	Duration
Isoniazid	*Adult*: 5 mg/kg	6 or 9 months daily
Isoniazid + Rifampicin	Isoniazid • *Adult*: 5 mg/kg • *Children*: 10 mg/kg • *Rifampicin*: Adults and children 10 mg/kg	3–4 months daily
Rifampicin	• *Adult*: 10 mg/kg • Children: 5 mg/kg	3–4 months daily

- Ongoing monitoring of CD4 counts and viral load is crucial, and any treatment changes should reflect these parameters.

Hepatitis B Infection

- In hepatitis-B positive patients, TNF-α inhibitors may be considered with concurrent antiviral therapy after a thorough risk-benefit evaluation.
- Guidelines recommend early treatment with nucleoside/nucleotide analogues of hepatitis B surface antigen (HBsAg)-positive patients requiring immunosuppressive therapies, starting prior to chemotherapy, and maintained for 6–12 months after completion of chemotherapy, as hepatitis B virus (HBV) may reactivate late after chemotherapy discontinuation.
  - Hepatitis B surface antigen +ve/anti-HBc +ve
    - Initiate anti-HBV prophylaxis before immunosuppressive or cytotoxic therapy.
    - Anti-HBV prophylaxis should be continued for at least *6–12 months* after completion of TNF-α inhibitors.
  - Hepatitis B surface antigen -ve/anti-HBc +ve
    - Regular monitoring for HBV DNA and liver function tests (LFT) (every 1–3 months) for on-demand therapy, continuing up to 12 months post-therapy cessation.
    - *Preferred drugs:* Entecavir, tenofovir

Hepatitis C Infection

Anti-TNF drugs in chronic hepatitis C patients are not contraindicated if monitoring of complete liver tests is performed every 3 months during treatment.

Monitoring

Pretreatment Evaluation

- *Clinical evaluation:* Specifically rule out infections especially tuberculosis, demyelinating disorders, and cardiac failure.
- Hemogram
- Liver and renal function tests (RFT)
- Evaluation for TB (chest X-ray, Mantoux/Quantiferon gold)

- Hepatitis B surface antigen, anti-HB surface Ab, anti-HB core Ab, and hepatitis C antibody tests
- Human immunodeficiency virus test

Follow-up Evaluation (Box 13.1)

- Blood tests [complete blood count (CBC), LFT, and RFT] every 3–6 months in patients who are prescribed TNF-α inhibitors without concomitant immunosuppressants and more frequent monitoring in patients who are prescribed concomitant immunosuppressants.
- Yearly testing for latent TB should be done in patients at high risk.[11] For patients who are not at high risk, screening should be done at the discretion of the dermatologist.

BOX 13.1 | **Tumor necrosis factor alpha (TNF-α) inhibitors.**

Baseline investigations:
- CBC with differential
- Liver and RFT
- Serological tests for hepatitis B and C and HIV
- *Tuberculosis (TB) screening:* Chest X-ray, purified protein derivative (PPD)/ Quantiferon gold
- *Heart failure evaluation:* Especially if there is a history or risk of congestive heart failure

Follow-up investigations:
- *Blood tests (CBC, LFT, and RFT):* Every 3–6 months
- *TB screening:* Annual for patients at high risk

Monitoring for adverse events:
- *Infections:* Increased risk within first 6–12 months, especially for TB
- *Injection/infusion reactions:* Manage based on severity
- *Demyelinating disease:* Look for neurological signs
- *Malignancies:* Screen for lymphoma/skin cancer
- *Heart failure:* Monitor for worsening heart failure symptoms

(CBC: complete blood count; LFT: liver function test; RFT: renal function test)

---

[11] Patients who are in contact with individuals with active TB and patients with selected underlying medical conditions.

Efficacy and Outcomes

- Tumor necrosis factor-alpha inhibitors typically demonstrate treatment efficacy within 12–16 weeks, except for infliximab, which may show results as early as 8–10 weeks.
- In clinical trials UNCOVER-2 and UNCOVER-3, etanercept achieved PASI 75 responses in 41.6–53.4% of patients, with PGA 0/1 outcomes in 36–41.6% at the 12-week mark.[12]
- Adalimumab, as indicated by meta-analysis, is potentially more effective than etanercept in reaching PASI 90, with BESURE trial data showing PASI 75 of 31.4% at week 4 and a PASI 90 of 47.7% and IGA 0/1 of 57.2 at week 16.[13]

Special Considerations

- Tumor necrosis factor-alpha inhibitors, classified as pregnancy category B, are generally deemed safe during pregnancy and breastfeeding.
- Infliximab, which crosses the placenta in the third trimester, does not appear to increase infection risks in infants during their first year, though cessation in the early third or late second trimester might limit placental transfer. These drugs are also considered safe for men planning to conceive.
- Neonates exposed to TNF inhibitors via maternal use should be considered immunocompromised for 1–3 months after birth. Regarding vaccinations, non-live vaccines are safe and effective for these infants, while live vaccines are contraindicated within the first 6 months postpartum.

Interleukin-17 Inhibitors

The IL-17 inhibitors approved for the management of psoriasis include secukinumab, ixekizumab, and brodalumab.

---

[12] Griffiths CE, Reich K, Lebwohl M, van de Kerkhof P, Paul C, Menter A, et al. Comparison of ixekizumab with etanercept or placebo in moderate-to-severe psoriasis (UNCOVER-2 and UNCOVER-3): results from two phase 3 randomised trials. Lancet. 2015;386(9993):541-51

[13] Thaçi D, Papp K, Marcoux D, Weibel L, Pinter A, Ghislain PD, et al. Sustained long-term efficacy and safety of adalimumab in paediatric patients with severe chronic plaque psoriasis from a randomized, double-blind, phase III study. Br J Dermatol. 2019;181(6):1177-89.

Chemical Structure

Secukinumab and ixekizumab are IgG1 monoclonal antibodies targeting IL-17A, whereas brodalumab is an IgG2 monoclonal antibody targeting the IL-17 receptor.

Mechanism of Action

These drugs inhibit the action of IL-17A or its receptor, crucial in the pathogenesis of psoriasis, leading to the reduction of pro-inflammatory cytokines and chemokines.

Pharmacokinetics

Secukinumab and ixekizumab reach peak serum concentrations several days post-dose, with steady state achieved by week 8 for ixekizumab and week 16 for secukinumab. Brodalumab reaches peak serum concentrations by approximately 3 days post-dose, with steady state achieved by week 4.

Indications

- Psoriasis (secukinumab and ixekizumab)
- Psoriatic arthritis (secukinumab and ixekizumab)

Contraindications

Absolute

- History of allergic reaction to the therapeutic agent or vehicle
- Inflammatory bowel disease (secukinumab and brodalumab).

Relative

- Active history or currently active inflammatory bowel disease (IBD)
- Suicidal ideation or behavior (brodalumab)

Available Formulations

- *Secukinumab:* 150 mg/mL prefilled syringe
- *Ixekizumab:* 80 mg/mL prefilled syringe
- *Brodalumab:* 210 mg/1.5 mL prefilled syringe

Dose and Administration

Refer to **Table 13.4**.

Adverse Effects

Common Side Effects

- Upper respiratory tract infections, headaches, dizziness, weariness, and loose stools are commonly seen side effects.
- Injection site pain and reactions occur in up to 20% of individuals receiving ixekizumab.
- Neutropenia is observed infrequently with both ixekizumab and brodalumab.

Mucocutaneous Candidiasis

- A higher rate of *Candida* infections is seen in patients using IL-17 inhibitors. Brodalumab has a higher occurrence rate (4%) compared to ixekizumab (3.3%) and secukinumab (1.7%). However, no instances of systemic candidiasis were identified in an analysis encompassing 21 clinical trials.
- Most *Candida* infections are mild-to-moderate and typically resolve with standard antifungal treatments without discontinuing the IL-17 inhibitors.

Inflammatory Bowel Disease

Patients with IBD (current or past) can have reactivation or aggravation of their condition.

TABLE 13.4: Dose and administration.

Biological agent	Loading dose	Maintenance
Secukinumab	300 mg subcutaneous injection at week 0, week 1, week 2, week 3, and week 4	300 mg subcutaneous injection every 4 weeks
Ixekizumab	160 mg subcutaneous injection followed by 80 mg on week 2, week 4, week 6, week 8, week 10, and week 12	80 mg subcutaneous injection every 4 weeks
Brodalumab	210-mg subcutaneous injection on week 0, week 1, and week 2	210 mg subcutaneous injection every 2 weeks

Suicidal Behavior

Reports indicate an increase in suicidal behavior among patients treated with IL-17 inhibitors, notably brodalumab, which has been linked to instances of suicide and is, therefore, not recommended for patients with current or past suicidal thoughts or actions.

Anti-drug Antibodies

A minority of secukinumab-treated patients developed anti-drug antibodies (ADAs), some of which were neutralizing, although these were often temporary and did not appear to impact the effectiveness or result in adverse events.

Mycobacterium Tuberculosis

Secukinumab is safe with respect to TB reactivation and may represent a good therapeutic option in patients with psoriasis and psoriatic arthritis who are at increased risk of TB.

Hepatitis B and C

Patients with currently active hepatitis B or C may receive an IL-17 inhibitor for the treatment of psoriasis. However, patients should first be evaluated and may require concomitant treatment with an approved antiviral medication directed against hepatitis B. The recommendations for screening and prophylaxis are similar to TNF-α antagonists.

Monitoring

Pretreatment Evaluation

- *Clinical evaluation:* Specifically rule out infections
- Hemogram
- Liver and RFT
- Rule out tuberculosis chest X-ray, PPD/Quantiferon gold.
- Serologic tests for hepatitis B and C, HIV

Follow-up Evaluation

- Follow-up visits can be scheduled from quarterly to twice yearly based on time of treatment, response, and tolerability of medication.

- During each visit patient should be assessed for:
  - Infections
  - Exacerbation/development of IBD
  - Monitoring for suicidal ideation is recommended for patients treated with brodalumab
  - Yearly testing for latent TB, as mentioned earlier for TNF-α blockers **(Box 13.2)**

Efficacy and Outcomes

The response to IL-17 inhibitors is assessed at 12 weeks, revealing secukinumab reaches PASI 75 in over 70% of patients, ixekizumab in 84.2%, and brodalumab between 85 and 86%.

Special Considerations

- Interleukin-17 inhibitors, while not extensively studied in human pregnancy, have demonstrated safety in animal studies;

BOX 13.2 **Interleukin (IL)-17 inhibitors.**

Baseline investigations:
- CBC with differential
- Liver and RFT
- Serological tests for hepatitis B and C and HIV
- *Tuberculosis (TB) screening:* Chest X-ray, purified protein derivative (PPD)/Quantiferon gold
- Mental health screening (if applicable)

Follow-up investigations:
- *Blood tests (CBC, LFT, RFT):* Every 3–6 months
- *TB screening:* Annual for patients at high risk

Monitoring for adverse events:
- *Infections:* Increased risk within first 6–12 months, especially for TB
- *Injection reactions:* Manage based on severity
- *Malignancies:* Screen for lymphoma/skin cancer
- *IBD symptoms:* Monitor for exacerbation
- *Mood changes:* Watch for mental health shifts

(CBC: complete blood count; IBD: inflammatory bowel disease; LFT: liver function test; RFT: renal function test)

secukinumab is categorized as pregnancy category B, indicating no observed harm to the developing fetus.

- Higher doses of ixekizumab or brodalumab than typically recommended have not shown fetal harm in animal studies, though an increase in neonatal deaths was noted, and these drugs have not been assigned a pregnancy category.
- Interleukin-17 inhibitors are considered potentially safe for use by men who are planning to conceive with their partners.

Interleukin-12/23 Inhibitors

The IL-12/23 inhibitors currently available for psoriasis treatment are ustekinumab, which target the shared p40 subunit of IL-12 and IL-23.

Chemical Structure

Ustekinumab is a human IgG1 kappa monoclonal antibody that binds to shared p40 subunit of IL-12 and IL-23.

Mechanism of Action

Ustekinumab binds to P40 subunit of both IL-12 and IL-23, thereby suppressing IL-12 and IL-23 mediated inflammation, resulting in inhibition of both Th1 and Th17 cells mediated inflammatory response in psoriasis.

Pharmacokinetics

- Median time to reach the maximum serum concentration (T_{max}) is approximately 13.5 days for a 45 mg dose and 7 days for a 90 mg dose in adults with psoriasis.
- Half-life elimination is 15–45 days.

Indications

- Adult and pediatric patients 6 years and older with moderate-to-severe plaque psoriasis who are candidates for phototherapy or systemic therapy.
- Psoriatic arthritis

Contraindications

Relative

- Untreated hepatitis B infection
- History of lymphoreticular malignancy
- Active infection (including TB) or sepsis. Initiation of therapy in patients with active infection should be done in consultation with an infectious disease specialist.

Absolute

History of allergic reaction to therapeutic agent or vehicle.

Available Formulations

Ustekinumab is available as a subcutaneous injection in single-dose prefilled syringes or vials at strengths of 45 mg/0.5 mL or 90 mg/mL.

Dose and Administration

- Adults weighing ≤100 kg should receive 45 mg subcutaneously initially, 4 weeks later, and then every 12 weeks.
- For adults >100 kg, the dose is 90 mg following the same schedule.

Adverse Events

- Common adverse events with ustekinumab include nasopharyngitis, upper respiratory tract infection, headache, and fatigue.
- There are rare reports of nonmelanoma skin cancers and reversible posterior leukoencephalopathy syndrome.

Monitoring

Pretreatment Evaluation

- *Clinical evaluation:* Specifically, for malignancy and active infections
- Hemogram
- Liver and RFT
- *Rule out tuberculosis:* Chest X-ray, PPD/Quantiferon gold.
- Serologic tests for hepatitis B, hepatitis C, and HIV.

Follow-up Evaluation (Box 13.3)

- Evaluate for infection, malignancy,[14] infusion/injection site reactions
- Complete blood count and LFT 3–6 monthly or as clinically indicated
- Yearly testing for latent TB should be done in patients at high risk

Efficacy and Outcomes

- Efficacy is apparent within 2 weeks, with 67% and 76% of patients reaching PASI 75 by week 12 on 45 mg and 90 mg doses, respectively, peaking between weeks 20 and 24.[15]
- Responses are sustained with continuous treatment for up to 1.5 years, and upon cessation, the median time to relapse is 15 weeks without rebound effects.

BOX 13.3 | **Interleukin (IL)-12/23 inhibitors.**

Baseline investigations:
- CBC with differential
- Liver and RFT
- Serological tests for hepatitis B and C and HIV
- *Tuberculosis (TB) screening:* Chest X-ray, purified protein derivative (PPD)/ Quantiferon gold

Follow-up investigations:
- *Blood tests (CBC, LFT, RFT):* Every 3–6 months
- *TB screening:* Annual for patients at high risk

Monitoring for adverse events:
- *Infections:* Increased risk within first 6–12 months, especially for TB
- *Injection site reactions:* Manage based on severity
- *Malignancies:* Screen for lymphoma/skin cancer
- *IBD exacerbation:* Look for GI symptoms

(CBC: complete blood count; IBD: inflammatory bowel disease; LFT: liver function test; RFT: renal function test)

---

[14] Specially for patients who has history of skin cancer.

[15] Papp KA, Langley RG, Lebwohl M, Krueger GG, Szapary P, Yeilding N, et al. Efficacy and safety of ustekinumab, a human interleukin-12/23 monoclonal antibody, in patients with psoriasis: 52-week results from a randomised, double-blind, placebo-controlled trial (PHOENIX 2). Lancet. 2008;371(9625):1675-84.

- Dose-response relationship exists but is not strictly linear; for partial responders, increasing the dosing frequency improves outcomes significantly on the 90 mg dose.
- Predictors of a poorer response include higher body weight, prior inadequate response to biologics, longer psoriasis duration, and the presence of psoriatic arthritis.

Special Considerations

- Ustekinumab is approved for plaque psoriasis in adolescents aged 12–17 years.
- Safety of ustekinumab during pregnancy and lactation is uncertain.

Interleukin-23 Inhibitors

Interleukin-23 inhibitors such as tildrakizumab and guselkumab are newer additions to the therapeutic arsenal against psoriasis, specifically targeting the IL-23 protein to help reduce the inflammation and skin cell turnover associated with the condition.

Chemical Structure

Both tildrakizumab and guselkumab are humanized monoclonal antibodies, with tildrakizumab being an IgG1/kappa and guselkumab an IgG1 lambda antibody.

Mechanism of Action

These drugs specifically target the p19 subunit of IL-23, preventing its interaction with the IL-23 receptor, which is integral to the inflammatory response in psoriasis.

Pharmacokinetics

Tildrakizumab has an estimated bioavailability of 73–80% post-subcutaneous injection, with a half-life of about 23 days.

Guselkumab displays linear pharmacokinetics with a mean steady-state trough serum concentration of approximately 1.2 µg/mL with a half-life of 18 days.

Indications

Indications for both include treatment of adults with moderate-to-severe plaque psoriasis who are candidates for systemic therapy or phototherapy.

Contraindications

Serious hypersensitivity to the active substances or any excipients is a contraindication for both medications.

Available Formulations

- *Tildrakizumab:* 100 mg/mL solution in single-dose prefilled syringes.
- *Guselkumab:* 100 mg/mL solution in prefilled syringes.

Dose and Administration

- The recommended dose for tildrakizumab is 100 mg at weeks 0, week 4, and then every 12 weeks.
- For guselkumab, it is 100 mg at week 0, week 4, and every 8 weeks thereafter.

Adverse Events

Common Adverse Reactions

- Common adverse reactions for both include upper respiratory infections and injection site reactions.
- Guselkumab may also cause headaches, arthralgia, diarrhea, gastroenteritis, tinea, and herpes simplex infections.

Reactions to Injection

Injection site reactions are among the commonly reported adverse effects for both drugs.

Formation of Antibodies

Approximately 6.5% of tildrakizumab-treated subjects and 6% of guselkumab-treated subjects developed antibodies to the respective drugs, with a subset being neutralizing antibodies which could potentially reduce efficacy.

Monitoring

Pretreatment Evaluation

- *Clinical evaluation:* Specifically, for malignancy and active infections
- Hemogram
- Liver and RFT
- *Rule out tuberculosis*: Chest X-ray, PPD/Quantiferon gold.
- Serologic tests for hepatitis B, hepatitis C, and HIV

Follow-up Evaluation (Box 13.4)

- Evaluate for infection, malignancy,[16] infusion/injection site reactions.
- Complete blood count and LFT 3–6 monthly or as clinically indicated.
- Yearly testing for latent TB should be done in patients at high risk.

BOX 13.4	Interleukin (IL)-23 inhibitors.

Baseline investigations:
- CBC with differential
- Liver and RFT
- Serological tests for hepatitis B and C and HIV
- *Tuberculosis (TB) screening:* Chest X-ray, purified protein derivative (PPD)/ Quantiferon gold

Follow-up investigations:
- *Blood tests (CBC, LFT, RFT):* Every 3–6 months
- *TB screening:* Annual for patients at high risk

Monitoring for adverse events:
- *Infections:* Increased risk within first 6–12 months, especially for TB
- *Injection/infusion reactions:* Manage based on severity
- *Demyelinating disease:* Look for neurological signs
- *Malignancies:* Screen for lymphoma/skin cancer
- *Heart failure:* Monitor for worsening heart failure symptoms

(CBC: complete blood count; LFT: liver function test; RFT: renal function test)

---

[16] Specially for patients who has history of skin cancer.

Efficacy and Outcomes

- The Phase 3 VOYAGE trials for guselkumab showed high efficacy, with 86–91% of patients achieving PASI 75 and 70–73% attaining PASI 90 by week 16.[17,18]
- The reSURFACE studies indicated tildrakizumab's efficacy with two-thirds of patients reaching PASI 75 and one-third achieving PASI 100 by week 12, which nearly doubled by week 28. The drug's efficacy is sustained over a long-term period of up to 5 years.[19]

Special Considerations

There is insufficient data on the use of both drugs in pregnant women. Animal studies have shown no harm to the developing fetus with secukinumab. In lactating monkeys, tildrakizumab was present in milk, but the safety and efficacy in pediatric patients have not been established for either drug.

---

[17] Blauvelt A, Papp KA, Griffiths CE, Randazzo B, Wasfi Y, Shen YK, et al. Efficacy and safety of guselkumab, an anti-interleukin-23 monoclonal antibody, compared with adalimumab for the continuous treatment of patients with moderate to severe psoriasis: results from the phase III, double-blinded, placebo and active comparator-controlled VOYAGE 1 trial. J Am Acad Dermatol. 2017;76(3):405-17.

[18] Reich K, Armstrong AW, Foley P, Song M, Wasfi Y, Randazzo B, et al. Efficacy and safety of guselkumab, an anti-interleukin-23 monoclonal antibody, compared with adalimumab for the treatment of patients with moderate to severe psoriasis with randomized withdrawal and retreatment: results from the phase III, double-blind, placebo- and active comparator-controlled VOYAGE 2 trial. J Am Acad Dermatol. 2017;76(3):418-31.

[19] Reich K, Warren RB, Iversen L, Puig L, Pau-Charles I, Igarashi A, et al. Long-term efficacy and safety of tildrakizumab for moderate-to-severe psoriasis: pooled analyses of two randomized phase III clinical trials (reSURFACE 1 and reSURFACE 2) through 148 weeks. Br J Dermatol. 2020;182(3):605-17.

Combination Therapy

Introduction

Though two or more drugs have been used for centuries in the management of psoriasis, it is only recently that formal protocols with multiple therapeutic agents have been devised.

Advantages of Combination Therapy

Recent data suggests several advantages of using multiple drugs in managing chronic, relapsing diseases like psoriasis:

- *Improved response*: Combinations of drugs may result in better and faster response, because different drugs act through different mechanisms—some agents act primarily on epidermal proliferation, others on the immunological mechanisms, while others through both pathways resulting in synergistic and additive efficacy.
- *Reduced toxicity*: Due to lower individual doses, reduced toxicity and side effects.

Protocols Used

The drugs can be used as:

- Conventional combination therapy
- Rotational therapy
- Sequential therapy

Conventional Combination Therapy

- Combination therapy involves simultaneous use of two or more agents (topical and/or systemic) with synergistic or complementary actions, e.g., when drugs A, B, and C are used at the same time.

- *Basis of combination*: Such a combination of drugs are used which:
  - Act in synergy resulting in faster and better clearance
  - Do not increase the side effects when used in combination. The maximum allowable dosage should not be exceeded for any of the drugs.
- *Factors determining switch to combination therapy*:
  - Poor response to monotherapy
  - Side effects (acute/chronic) to drug used
  - Comorbidities precluding maximum prescribable dose
- *Factors determining the choice of combination*:
  - Severity of disease
  - Patient's expectations
  - Ease of use
  - History related to use of agents in the combination:
    - Response
    - Side effects
  - Cost
  - Comorbidities in the patient
- *Common combinations used*: Some drugs used in psoriasis are compatible, while others should not be used simultaneously **(Table 14.1)**. Combinations frequently used include:
  - *For localized lesions [< 10% body surface area (BSA)]:* A combination of topical agents are generally used both for synergistic action as well as for enhancing penetration and improving response. The frequently used combinations in topical therapy include:
    - *Steroids + salicylic acid in ointment base:* Wherein salicylic acid improves efficacy of steroids by virtue of its kerato-lytic action.
    - *Steroids + calcipotriol in ointment base:* Wherein both steroids and calcipotriol are effective in psoriasis, calcipotriol also acts as steroid-sparing agent while steroids reduce irritation of calcipotriol.
    - Coal tar + salicylic acid in ointment base.
  - *For widespread disease (>10% BSA):* A combination of one or two systemic agents or a systemic agent with ultraviolet

TABLE 14.1: Compatibility of different topical and systemic agents used in psoriasis.

	CT	Dith	Cst	T	Cal	Mtx	Aci	CsA	NB-UVB	PUVA
Topical agents										
Coal tar (CT)	X	++	+	?	+	+	+	+	++	-*
Dithranol (Dith)	++	X	+	?	+	+	+	+	++	+
Steroids (Cst)	+	+	X	++	++	+	+	+	+	+
Tazarotene (T)	+	+	++	X	+	+	+	+	++	++
Calcipotriol (Cal)	+	+	++	+	X	+	++	+++	++**	++**
Systemic agents										
Methotrexate (Mtx)	+	+	+	+	+	X	-***	??	-	-
Acitretin (Aci)	+	+	+	+	++	-	X	4-	++	++-****
Cyclosporine A (CsA)	+	+	+	+	++	-	-	X	-	
Photo/Photochemotherapy										
NB-UVB	++	++	+	++	++**	-	++	-	X	-
PUVA	-*	+	+	++	++**	-	++	-****	-	X

*Causes phototoxicity.

**Calcipotriol to be used after photoexposure.

***Causes hepatotoxicity.

****Increased incidence of neoplasms.

(NB-UVB: narrow band ultraviolet B; PUVA: psoralen with ultraviolet A)

B (UVB) or psoralen with ultraviolet A (PUVA) are used invariably in combination with a topical agent. The aim is to obtain better, faster, and safer therapeutic response. Apparent synergistic enhancement is seen with many of the combinations used. The frequently used combinations in systemic therapy include:

- *Acitretin + PUVA (RePUVA) + topical therapy:* Wherein acitretin improves penetration of UVA because of its effect on keratinization and acitretin protects against carcinogenic potential of PUVA.
- *Acitretin + UVB (ReUVB) + topical therapy:* Wherein acitretin improves penetration of UVA because of its effect on keratinization and acitretin protects against carcinogenic potential of UVB.
- Cyclosporine and methotrexate
- Methotrexate + UVB
- *Cyclosporine + PUVA:* Contraindicated because of increased risk of cancer

Rotational Therapy

- *Definition*: Rotational therapy involves utilizing a highly effective, but "potentially toxic" monotherapy for a specific (fixed) period of time and then switching to a less effective but safer therapy. Initially, the concept of rotational therapy started using rotation of UVB + tar, PUVA, methotrexate, and retinoids but has now been expanded to include other systemic agents like cyclosporine.
- *Basis:* It is done basically to minimize cumulative dose and forestall toxicities. Also to overcome problem of tachyphylaxis,[1] which is seen with some medications like topical corticosteroids.
- *Indications:* More commonly used in the treatment of severe psoriasis which warrants use of potentially toxic systemic agents such as methotrexate, cyclosporine, or oral retinoids. This strategy may be resorted to at the beginning of therapy or based on patient's response or development of side effects.

---

[1] *Tachyphylaxis*: Reduced response to therapy with continued use.

- *When to rotate*:
  - *Fixed intervals*: At fixed intervals (e.g., 6/12/24 months)
  - *Patient's response*: When patient remits, switch to less effective, safe therapy and when patient flares, switch to more effective but toxic therapy.
  - *Side effects*: When agent being used is ineffective, is producing intolerable side effects or the cumulative dose of agent being used approaches toxicity.
- *Choice of next agent:* Depends on:
  - Side effects, produced by current therapy
  - Cost factors
  - Comorbidities present in patient
  - Outcome expected by patient
  - Past medications and response
- *Agents used* **(Table 14.2)***:* Both topical and systemic agents are used in rotational therapy. Patients are treated initially with primary agents and switched to secondary agents, if:
  - Primary agents are ineffective
  - Unacceptable side effects or cumulative toxicity develops to primary agents.

Sequential Therapy

- *Basis*: It is designed to optimize initial efficacy followed by safe maintenance regimen by using specific combinations of topical agents, (for mild-to-moderate psoriasis) or systemic agents and/ or phototherapy for severe psoriasis in a deliberate sequence.

TABLE 14.2: Agents used in rotational therapy.

Primary agents	Secondary agents	Low dose combinations
• Methotrexate • Acitretin • PUVA • PUVA sol • UVB +/– tar • Cyclosporine	• Hydroxyurea • Sulfasalazine	• Hydroxyurea (< 1 g/day) + PUVA + topicals • Methotrexate (< 10 mg/week) + topicals • Retinoids + PUVA sol + topicals • Cyclosporine (< 3 mg/kg/day) + methotrexate (< 10 mg/week) + topicals

(PUVA: psoralen with ultraviolet A; UVB: ultraviolet B)

- *Steps*: It consists of three steps:
  1. *Clearing phase:* It involves the use of a powerful, rapid-acting agent, (often "toxic"/expensive) such as cyclosporine at maximum dose.
  2. *Transitional phase:* A phase in which a well-tolerated, safe maintenance drug is administered concurrently with the clearing agent which is gradually tapered.
  3. *Maintenance phase*: A phase in which the patient is on maintenance therapy, usually with one agent, sometimes with more.
- *Regimens used:*
  - Regimen for resource-poor settings **(Table 14.3)**.
  - Standard regimen **(Table 14.4)**

TABLE 14.3: Sequential therapy for resource poor settings.

Clearing phase (1–3 m)	Methotrexate (15–25 mg weekly)
Transition phase (4–6 m)	Methotrexate (7.5 mg weekly) + acitretin (25 mg daily)[*]
Maintenance phase (>6 m)	Acitretin (25 mg daily) + PUVA sol

[*] Methotrexate and acitretin: Keeping a close watch on liver function tests (and hematological parameters).

(PUVA: psoralen with ultraviolet A)

TABLE 14.4: Commonly used sequential therapy acitretin.

Clearing phase	Transition phase		Maintenance phase
Month 0–1: CsA (5 mg/kg/day)	*Months 2–7*: Introduce acitretin at 25 mg and uptitrate by 10 mg monthly until maximally tolerated dose	• CsA taper 1 mg/kg/ month • Maintain with acitretin	*Month 7 onward*: • Maintain on acitretin • Add UVB or PUVA if necessary

(CsA: cyclosporine A; PUVA: psoralen with ultraviolet A; UVB: ultraviolet B)

Approach to a Patient with Psoriasis

Introduction

A patient presenting for the first time with psoriasis expects a positive yet sympathetic response from the treating physician. He also needs to be adequately clinically evaluated before treatment is initiated.

History

Complete history is taken and preferably recorded in a proforma **(Annexure 1)**. The history should include:

- Duration of disease
- Onset and course of disease
- History of nail and joint involvement
- History of erythroderma and episodes of pustulation
- *Exacerbating factors*: Season (winter or summer aggravation), stress, trauma, photoexposure,[1] alcohol, smoking, and drugs [beta blockers, lithium, nonsteroidal anti-inflammatory drugs (NSAIDs), corticosteroids, and antimalarials].
- Evaluation of effect of disease on physical, emotional, and social aspects of patient's life, i.e., effect of psoriasis on patient's quality of life. For this a dermatology life quality index (DLQI) could be used. Or a psoriasis specific instrument may be used **(Annexure 2)**.
- Past and current treatments taken and response thereof.
- Other diseases, e.g., diabetes, hypertension, and related treatment taken.

---

[1] *Photoaggravated psoriasis*: Such lesions will be seen on photoexposed parts and phototherapy/photochemotherapy is preferably avoided.

Examination

Examination includes the following discussed here.

Evaluation of Disease

A proforma may be used to note the following parameters **(Annexure 1)**:

- *Type of psoriasis*: Chronic plaque/guttate/erythroderma/generalized pustular/palmoplantar pustulosis
- Percentage of body surface area (BSA) involved and whether sites like palms, soles, scalp, and face are affected.
- Nail changes and joint involvement
- To evaluate severity of psoriasis, joint, and nail involvement **(Annexure 3)**

Further Evaluation of Patient

The following should be specifically evaluated in patients:

- Anemia, status of liver, and joint involvement
- Evaluation of effect of disease on physical, emotional, and social aspects of patient's life, i.e., effect of psoriasis on patient's quality of life **(Annexure 2)**.
- Evaluation for comorbidities

Information to Patient

It is necessary to discuss the disease with the patients **(Annexure 4)**.

Treatment Options Available (Flowcharts 15.1 to 15.3)

The choice of treatment depends on several factors:

- Clinical severity of disease on skin, joints, and nails:
  - Mild disease (BSA < 2%) is best treated with topical agents. Moderately severe disease (BSA 2–10%) is initially treated with topical agents, failing which photo/photochemotherapy and systemic agents are added. For severe disease (BSA >10%), treatment is initiated unless contraindicated with

photo/photochemotherapy or with systemic therapy with topical therapy(ies) being used as adjuvant.

- Nail psoriasis if severe enough and impacting patient's quality of life (QoL) warrants systemic therapy and so also joint involvement.
- Impact of disease on the patient's QoL
- Comorbidities
- Cost constraints

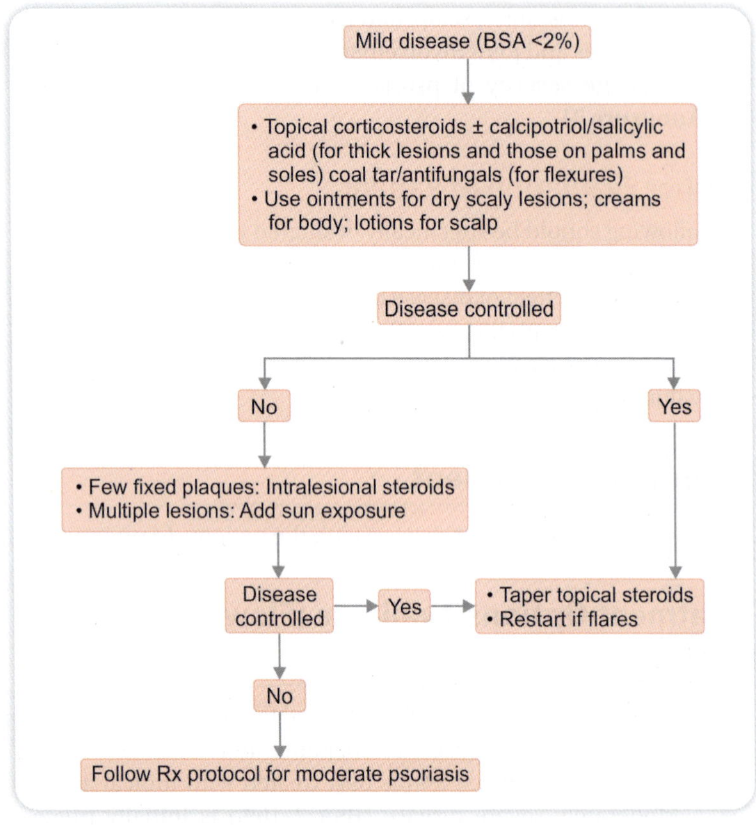

Flowchart 15.1: Treatment protocol for mild psoriasis [body surface area (BSA) < 2%].

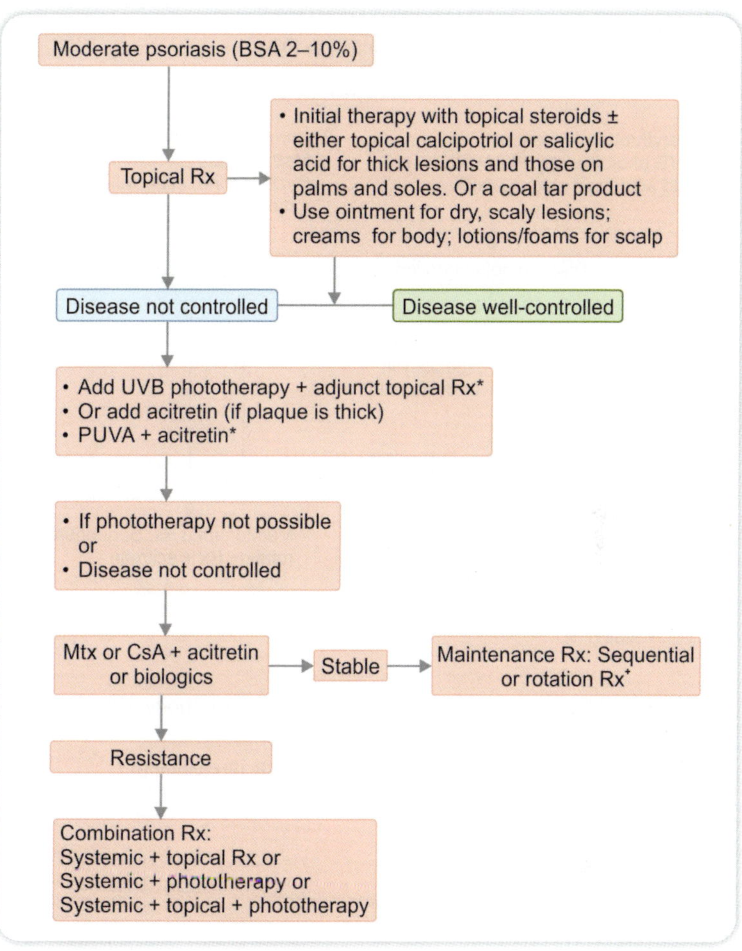

* Refer Chapter 10 Topical Therapy
\+ Refer Chapter 14 Combination Therapy

Flowchart 15.2: Treatment protocol for moderate psoriasis [body surface area (BSA) 2–10%].

(CsA: cyclosporine A; Mtx: methotrexate; PUVA: psoralen with ultraviolet A; UVB: ultraviolet B)

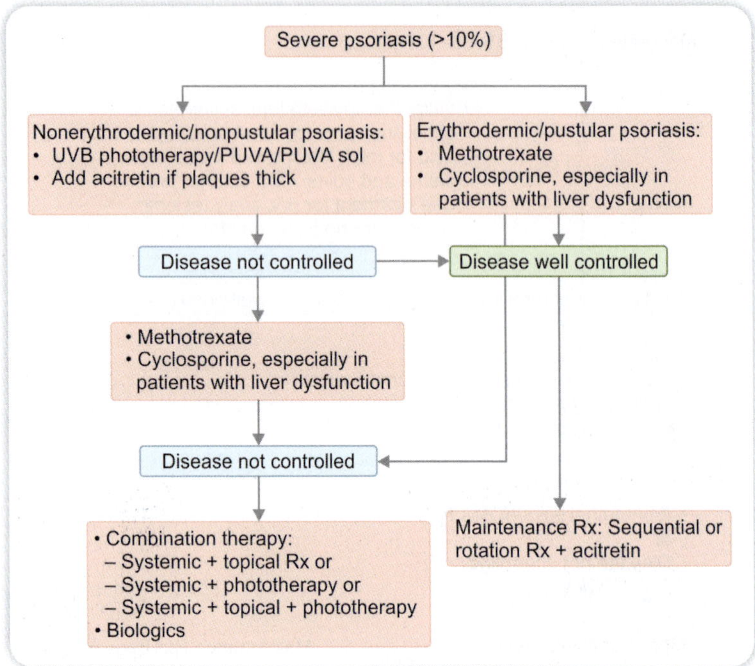

Flowchart 15.3: Treatment protocol for severe psoriasis [body surface area (BSA) >10%].

(PUVA: psoralen with ultraviolet A; UVB: ultraviolet B)

Section 3

Annexures

Annexures

ANNEXURE 1

Proforma for Psoriasis Patients

Name: _____________________________   Age/Sex: __________

Marital status: _________________   Occupation: _________________

Address:_________________________   Income: _________________

____

History

Chief complaints with duration:

Course of disease and site(s) of onset:

- Itchy/nonitchy
- History of Koebnerization
- Seasonal change
- Spontaneous remission
- Any triggers for recent exacerbation-drugs/fever/sore throat/ discontinuing treatment/alternative medicine/seasonal variation

History of Complications

	Number of episodes and duration of each	Total duration in weeks
Erythroderma		
Pustular lesions		

History of Associations

	Duration	Type
Nail changes		
Joint pains—which joints/morning stiffness/swelling/deformity/functional disability		

History of Previous Treatment with Response

	Treatment	Duration	Response
1.			
2.			
3.			
4.			

History of

Disease	Duration	Comments	Treatment
Hypertension			
Diabetes mellitus			
Tuberculosis			
Cardiac disease			
Liver disease			
Renal disease			
Others			

Family History

Disease	Yes/No	Comments
Psoriasis		
Hypertension		
Diabetes mellitus		
Tuberculosis		
Cardiac disease		

Personal History

	Nonsmoker	Ex-smoker			Current smoker	
Smoking		Quantity/day	Duration	Stopped since (month)	Quantity/day	Duration
	Nondrinker	Ex-drinker			Current drinker	
Alcohol		Quantity/day	Duration	Stopped since (month)	Quantity/day	Duration

Examination

General Physical Examination

Pallor/edema/cyanosis/clubbing/lymphadenopathy/icterus:

- *Weight*: kg
- *Height*: m
- *BMI*: kg/m^2
- *Waist circumference*: cm
- *Pulse rate*:
- *BP*:

Mucocutaneous Examination

- Distribution
- Type of lesions—guttate lesions/plaques/pustular/erythroderma
- Auspitz sign
- Palm/sole/scalp/genital/flexures involvement
- BSA
- PASI

Nail Changes

	Numbers RL		Changes seen	Comments
Fingernails			Pitting/oil drop/plate thickening/onycholysis/subungual hyperkeratosis/discoloration	
Toe nails			Pitting/oil drop/plate thickening/onycholysis/subungual hyperkeratosis/discoloration	

Joint Involvement

Site	UL	Elbow/wrist/MCP/IP
	LL	Knee/Ankle/MTP/IP
	Axial	Spine + Sacroiliac joint or spine alone or sacroiliac joint alone
Type of joint		Small joints/large joints
Number(s)		1 or >1
Symmetry		Symmetrical/asymmetrical
Associating with		Swelling/restriction of joints/digital foreshortening/tenderness
Deformity		
Comments		Classical/oligoarthritis/RA factor-negative polyarthritis/Arthritis mutilans/Axial arthritis

Systemic Examination

- Cardiovascular
- Chest
- Abdomen
- Any other

Diagnosis:
- Plaque/pustular/erythrodermic/guttate
- Arthropathy
- Nail involvement
- Metabolic syndrome
- Other comorbidities
- BSA
- PASI

Investigations

Date					
Hemogram: • Hb • TLC • DLC • Platelet • ESR					
RFT: • Urea • Creatinine					
LFT: • Bil • SGOT/SGPT/ALP *Lipid profile:* • Total cholesterol • TG • HDL-C • LDL-C					
Urine: • RE • ME					
ECG					
Radiological evaluation: • Chest X-ray • Joints					

Treatment and Follow-up

Coal tar/Topical steroids/Calcipotriol/Anthralin/Any other PUVAsol/PUVA/NB UVB

MTX/ Cys A/Acitretin/Isotretinoin/Any other (Biologicals)

Date	Treatment	Response	Adverse effects

ANNEXURE 2

Quality of Life Measures

Several measures, either dermatology specific or psoriasis specific can be used to evaluate the impact of psoriasis on patients' life, quality of life (QOL).

Dermatology Life Quality Index

- Dermatology Life Quality Index is a dermatology-specific quality of life questionnaire used in adults with evidenced reliability and validity.
- It is a good index to use, if one has to compare disability caused by one dermatological condition versus another.
- Dermatology Life Quality Index contains 10 questions under six domains concerning patients' perception of effect of their skin disease on various aspects of their life, including symptoms and feelings (questions 1 and 2), daily activities (questions 3 and 4), leisure and sports (questions 5 and 6), work or school (question 7), personal relationships (questions 8 and 9), and treatment (question 10).
- All questions relate to the previous week, with each question answered according to intensity of impact.
- Responses are precoded (0 = not at all, 1 = a little, 2 = a lot, 3 = very much) and the DLQI is calculated by summing the score of each question, resulting in a maximum of 30 and a minimum of 0. Higher the score, more the impairment of QOL.

Psoriasis Disability Index

- Psoriasis Disability Index (PDI) is an appropriate method to give a rapid global measure of psoriasis disability, as it refers to impact of psoriasis on daily activities, work, personal relationships, leisure, and treatment-related aspects based on previous 4 weeks.
- The questionnaire includes 15 questions and respondents rate questions on a 7-point linear analogue, ranging from "0" (no disability) to "6" (maximum disability).

<u>**DERMATOLOGY LIFE QUALITY INDEX**</u>

DLQI

Hospital No: Date: Score:

Name:

Address: Diagnosis:

The aim of this questionnaire is to measure how much your skin problem has affected your life OVER THE LAST WEEK. Please tick ☑ one box for each question.

1. Over the last week, how **itchy**, **sore**, **painful** or **stinging** has your skin been?
   - Very much ☐
   - A lot ☐
   - A little ☐
   - Not at all ☐

2. Over the last week, how **embarrassed** or **self conscious** have you been because of your skin?
   - Very much ☐
   - A lot ☐
   - A little ☐
   - Not at all ☐

3. Over the last week, how much has your skin interfered with you going **shopping** or looking after your **home** or **garden**?
   - Very much ☐
   - A lot ☐
   - A little ☐
   - Not at all ☐   Not relevant ☐

4. Over the last week, how much has your skin influenced the **clothes** you wear?
   - Very much ☐
   - A lot ☐
   - A little ☐
   - Not at all ☐   Not relevant ☐

5. Over the last week, how much has your skin affected any **social** or **leisure** activities?
   - Very much ☐
   - A lot ☐
   - A little ☐
   - Not at all ☐   Not relevant ☐

6. Over the last week, how much has your skin made it difficult for you to do any **sport**?
   - Very much ☐
   - A lot ☐
   - A little ☐
   - Not at all ☐   Not relevant ☐

7. Over the last week, has your skin prevented you from **working** or **studying**?
   - Yes ☐
   - No ☐   Not relevant ☐

   If "No", over the last week how much has your skin been a problem at **work** or **studying**?
   - A lot ☐
   - A little ☐
   - Not at all ☐

8. Over the last week, how much has your skin created problems with your **partner** or any of your **close friends** or **relatives**?
   - Very much ☐
   - A lot ☐
   - A little ☐
   - Not at all ☐   Not relevant ☐

9. Over the last week, how much has your skin caused any **sexual difficulties**?
   - Very much ☐
   - A lot ☐
   - A little ☐
   - Not at all ☐   Not relevant ☐

10. Over the last week, how much of a problem has the **treatment** for your skin been, for example by making your home messy, or by taking up time?
    - Very much ☐
    - A lot ☐
    - A little ☐
    - Not at all ☐   Not relevant ☐

Please check you have answered EVERY question. Thank you.

Source: Finlay AY, Khan GK. Dermatology Life Quality Index (DLQI)—a simple practical measure for routine clinical use. Clinical and Experimental Dermatology. 1994;19(3):210-6.

त्वचारोग जीवन गुणवत्ता सूची · डीएलक्यूआई

अस्पताल क्रमांक :   दिनांक :   स्कोर :

नाम :   रोग निदान :

पता :

इस प्रश्नोत्तरी का उद्देश्य यह नापना है कि आपकी त्वचा की परेशानी ने गत सप्ताह में आपके जीवन पर कितना प्रभाव डाला है. कृपया हर प्रश्न के लिए एक बाक्स में टिक करें.

१.	गत् सप्ताह, आपकी त्वचा में कितनी **खुजली, पीड़ा, दर्द** या **चुभन** लग रहा था?	बहुत ज्यादा ☐ बहुत ☐ थोड़ा ☐ बिलकुल नहीं ☐	
२.	गत् सप्ताह, अपनी त्वचा के कारण आप कितने **शर्मसार** या **स्व चैतन्य** हुए?	बहुत ज्यादा ☐ बहुत ☐ थोड़ा ☐ बिलकुल नहीं ☐	
३.	गत् सप्ताह, आपकी त्वचा ने आपकी **खरीदारी, घर या गार्डन** की देखभाल के काम पर कितना प्रभाव डाला?	बहुत ज्यादा ☐ बहुत ☐ थोड़ा ☐ बिलकुल नहीं ☐	लागू नहीं ☐
४.	गत् सप्ताह, आपकी त्वचा ने आपके **कपड़े** पहनने पर कितना प्रभाव डाला?	बहुत ज्यादा ☐ बहुत ☐ थोड़ा ☐ बिलकुल नहीं ☐	लागू नहीं ☐
५.	गत् सप्ताह, आपकी त्वचा ने आपके **सामाजिक जीवन** या **फुर्सत के समय** की गतिविधियों पर कितना प्रभाव डाला?	बहुत ज्यादा ☐ बहुत ☐ थोड़ा ☐ बिलकुल नहीं ☐	लागू नहीं ☐
६.	गत् सप्ताह, आपकी त्वचा ने आपके **खेलकूद** के लिए कितनी मुश्किलें खड़ी कीं?	बहुत ज्यादा ☐ बहुत ☐ थोड़ा ☐ बिलकुल नहीं ☐	लागू नहीं ☐
७.	गत् सप्ताह, आपकी त्वचा ने आपके **काम** या **पढ़ाई** में कोई रुकावट डाली?	हां ☐ नहीं ☐	लागू नहीं ☐
	इसका उत्तर अगर नहीं है, तो गत् सप्ताह आपकी त्वचा ने आपके **काम** या **पढ़ाई** में कितनी परेशानी खड़ी की ?	बहुत ☐ थोड़ा ☐ बिलकुल नहीं ☐	
८.	गत सप्ताह, आपकी त्वचा ने आपके **पार्टनर** या किसी भी **करीबी मित्र** या **रिश्तेदार** के लिए कितनी परेशानी खड़ी की	बहुत ज्यादा ☐ बहुत ☐ थोड़ा ☐ बिलकुल नहीं ☐	लागू नहीं ☐
९.	गत् सप्ताह, आपकी त्वचा के कारण कितनी **सेक्सुअल मुश्किलें** आईं?	बहुत ज्यादा ☐ बहुत ☐ थोड़ा ☐ बिलकुल नहीं ☐	लागू नहीं ☐
१०.	गत सप्ताह, आपकी त्वचा के **उपचार** ने आपके लिए कितनी मुश्किलें बढ़ाई, उदाहरण के लिए घर को अस्त–व्यस्त बनाना, या समय का नुकसान करना.	बहुत ज्यादा ☐ बहुत ☐ थोड़ा ☐ बिलकुल नहीं ☐	लागू नहीं ☐

कृपया देख लें कि आपने हर प्रश्न का उत्तर दे दिया है. धन्यवाद.

ENGLISH TO HINDI
18 JANUARY 2008

Source: Finlay AY, Khan GK. Dermatology Life Quality Index (DLQI)--a simple practical measure for routine clinical use. Clinical and Experimental Dermatology. 1994;19(3):210-6.

ANNEXURE 3

Clinical Severity Assessment

Several scores are available for assessing severity of psoriasis including:

- Body surface area (BSA)
- Psoriasis area and severity index (PASI)
- Psoriasis global assessment (PGA)
- Self-administered psoriasis area and severity index
- Nail psoriasis severity index
- Severity of joint involvement

Body Surface Area

- Simplest scoring system
- Does not reflect severity of disease, but only body surface area involved
- Follows rule of nine

Psoriasis Area and Severity Index

- Most frequently used instrument for new drug evaluation
- Cumbersome, taking about 10 minutes/patient
- Area, erythema, induration, and scaling graded and multiplied by a factor which is 0.1 for head, 0.2 for upper extremities, 0.3 for trunk and 0.4 for lower extremities.

Psoriasis Area and Severity Index

	Area	Erythema	Induration	Scaling
Head (h)				
Upper ext (u)				
Trunk (t)				
Lower ext (l)				
Total				

$$PASI = 0.1(E_h + I_h + S_h) A_h + 0.2 (E_u + I_u + S_u) A_u +$$
$$0.3 (E_t + I_t + S_t) A_t + 0.4 (E_l + I_l + S_l) A_l$$

Where, E = erythema, I = induration, S = scaling, A = area

Area scoring		Erythema, induration, and scaling	
Score	% involvement	Score	
1	<10%	0	None
2	11–30%	1	Slight
3	31–50%	2	Moderate
4	51–70%	3	Severe
5	71–90%	4	Extraordinarily severe
6	91–100%		

Psoriasis Global Assessment

- Most often employed scoring system used in clinical trials to measure psoriasis severity
- Quicker than PASI, but less objective
- Investigator assigns a single instrument of patient overall severity disease—typically, a 7-point scale from clear-to-severe is used, although many variations have been employed. Possible scores are:
  - *Cleared*: 100% improvement; no sign of psoriasis (post-inflammatory hyperpigmentation may be present)
  - *Almost clear*: 75–99% improvement; intermediate between cleared and mild
  - *Mild*: 50–74% improvement; slight plaque elevation, scaling, and/or erythema
  - *Mild-to-moderate*: 25–49% improvement; intermediate between moderate-and-mild
  - *Moderate*: 1–24% improvement; moderate plaque elevation, scaling, and/or erythema
  - *Moderate-to-severe*: Marked plaque elevation, scaling, and/or erythema
  - *Severe*: Very marked plaque elevation, scaling, and/or erythema
- All these groups can be utilized with different descriptions and scores; even if the individual elements of psoriasis plaque morphology or degree of body surface area involvement are not quantified.

Self-administered Psoriasis Area Severity Index

- It is a clinical instrument used to measure extent of psoriasis on the body surface.
- Index may be filled by physician or patient. Respondents shade affected areas in a silhouette representing the front and back of human body and rate erythema, thickness, and scaliness of an average lesion on separate visual analogue scales (VASs). Finally, the scores are entered into a formula to produce an overall severity score. The range and interpretation of Self-Administered Psoriasis Area Severity Index (SAPASI) scores are similar to those of PASI.

Nail Psoriasis Severity Index

- It is a simple tool used to evaluate nail psoriasis, with a score 4 being given to nail bed and nail matrix psoriasis, for each nail.
- Nail plate is divided into four quadrants (by an imaginary longitudinal and horizontal line) and assessed in each quadrant for:
  - Nail matrix psoriasis, i.e., nail pitting, leukonychia, red spots in lunula, and crumbling.
  - Nail bed psoriasis, i.e., onycholysis, oil drop (salmon patch) dyschromia, splinter hemorrhage, and subungual hyperkeratosis.

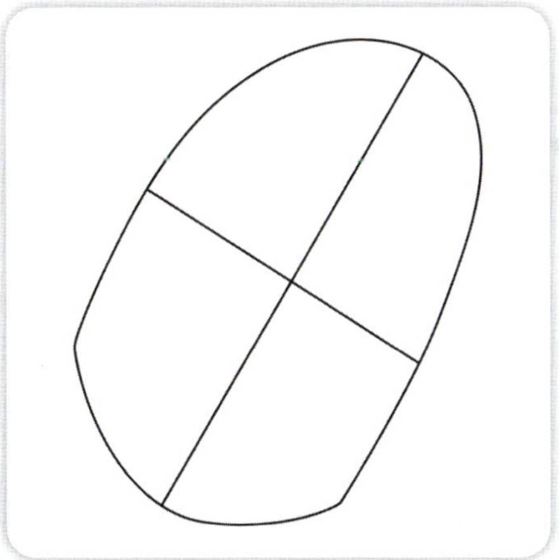

- Lesions are scored as:
  - 0, if findings are absent.
  - 1, if present in 1 quadrant of nail.
  - 2, if present in 2 quadrants of nail.
  - 3, if present in 3 quadrants of nail.
  - 4, if present in all quadrants of nail.
- Nail score is sum of nail matrix and nail bed scores (0–4 each) and Nail Psoriasis Severity Index (NAPSI) is total score of all involved nails.
- For a more sensitive scale, each nail can be given a separate score for all eight features in each quadrant. The resulting score then is a 0–32 scale for each nail.

Scoring of Psoriatic Arthritis

American College of Rheumatology (ACR) is a complex score, including a number of joints affected, patient's assessment of disease activity, disability and pain, physician's global assessment, and laboratory variables such as ESR and CRP. A simpler score is the disease activity score (DAS or DAS28), which includes the number of swollen and tender joints (maximum of 28), C-reactive protein, PGA, and VAS. Improvements in ACR or DAS of 20% or more are considered as significant, implying only reversible damage in arthritis.

ANNEXURE 4
Patient Information on Psoriasis

What is Psoriasis?

- Psoriasis is a common noncontagious skin condition.
- It is characterized by presence of red, thick scaly patches of different sizes and shapes.

What are the Symptoms?

Lesions of psoriasis can be itchy. Some patients (about 10%) with psoriasis also have joint pains and swelling.

What are the Associations of Psoriasis?

Psoriasis can involve the nails and joints. Usually there are no systemic associations, but recent studies have shown a greater association of obesity, high blood pressure, diabetes, and increased levels of cholesterol and triglycerides in patients with psoriasis.

What Happens to Joints in Psoriasis?

- About 10% of patients with psoriasis have joint involvement in the form of *psoriatic arthritis*. Although the joints of the hands, knees, and ankles are most commonly involved, almost any joint can be involved. Psoriatic arthritis is treated with medications to stop disease progression.
- Joint involvement usually follows skin involvement but may precede it. Sometimes joint pain and swelling may be the only sign of psoriasis with no lesions on skin.
- Average age for onset of psoriatic arthritis is 30–40 years of age.
- The diagnosis of psoriatic arthritis is typically made by examination, medical history, and relevant family history. Sometimes laboratory tests and X-rays may be used to determine the severity of the disease and to exclude other diagnoses such as rheumatoid arthritis and osteoarthritis.

What is the Association between Nails and Psoriasis?

- Psoriasis affects the nails in about 50% of patients.
- Nails may have small pinpoint pits or large yellowish separations of the nail plate called "oil spots."
- Nail psoriasis is often difficult to treat as treatment options are limited and include potent topical steroids applied at the nail-base cuticle, injection of steroids at the nail-base cuticle, and oral or systemic medications for treatment of psoriasis.

Is Psoriasis Contagious?

No, psoriasis is not contagious. It is not spread by touching, speaking, sitting, or sharing utensils of persons with psoriasis.

Is it Genetic?

Though genetic factors do play a role in psoriasis, their exact role has not been defined. Though there is a greater chance of blood relatives of patients who have psoriasis to develop the disease, most patients with psoriasis themselves do not have a family history of psoriasis.

Can a Person with Psoriasis Marry?

Yes, a person with psoriasis can marry. And since the disease is not contagious, it will not be transmitted to the spouse.

Will Psoriasis Interfere with My Employment?

No, it will not.

What Causes Psoriasis?

- The exact cause is unknown.
- It probably develops due to a combination of factors, including genetic predisposition and environmental factors.
- The immune system plays a major role but what triggers the disease has still not been found.

Is it Caused or Aggravated by Any Food?

No, it is not aggravated by any food, but sometimes excessive alcohol consumption and smoking may trigger it.

What is the Course of Psoriasis?

- Psoriasis is considered as long-term (chronic) skin condition.
- It has a variable course of periodic improvement and worsening. It is like fever—once you have recovered from a bout, there is no guarantee that you will not get fever again.
- Sometimes psoriasis may clear for years and the patient will remain well.
- Most people have worsening of disease in winter with improvement in summer or with increased sunlight exposure.

Who can get Psoriasis?

- Anybody can get psoriasis. Psoriasis is seen worldwide, in all races and both sexes.
- Though there is a greater chance of "blood relatives" of patients who have psoriasis to develop the disease, most patients with psoriasis themselves do not have a family history of psoriasis.
- Though it can be seen in people of any age from cradle to grave, most patients first develop the disease in their early 20s.

Which Parts of the Body can be Involved?

- Though any part of the skin can be affected, psoriasis classically affects skin over elbows, knees, and lower back, areas which are prone to trauma. Scalp is another common site of involvement.
- In a few patients, disease can be generalized, wherein virtually the entire body is fully covered with thick red, scaly skin. This is called erythroderma.
- Psoriasis can involve the nails most frequently in form of the very small pits (pinpoint depressions or white spots on the nail) or as larger yellowish-brown separations of the nail bed called "oil spots." Nail psoriasis is often incorrectly diagnosed as a fungal infection.

How is Psoriasis Diagnosed?

Diagnosis of psoriasis is generally made on the basis of the look of the patches. Sometimes a biopsy may be needed to establish the diagnosis.

Can it be Life-threatening?

Psoriasis by itself is NOT a life-threatening condition. Some patients develop complications such as pustules and generalized psoriasis (erythroderma) and these may be associated with complications.

What are the Available Treatment Options for Psoriasis?

While psoriasis cannot be cured, it can be controlled, and we have several options available to do so. The patient's health, age, lifestyle, and the severity of psoriasis determine which treatment options are appropriate. In most patients, a combination of drugs is used either simultaneously or sequentially or in rotation.

Depending on the extent of disease, different forms of treatment are used:

- *For localized lesions,* topical treatment is used:
  - Coal tar
  - Dithranol
  - Topical steroids with/without salicylic acid
  - Topical retinoids
- *For extensive lesions,* oral (rarely injectable) medications and/or light treatment is used:
  - Narrow band UVB
  - PUVA/PUVA sol
  - Methotrexate
  - Acitretin
  - Cyclosporine
  - Apremilast
  - Biologicals

How is Coal Tar Used?

Coal tar is produced by destructive distillation of coal. It has been used for more than a century, to safely and effectively treat psoriasis. Coal tar is messy to use but today's products are greatly improved and less messy.

When are (Cortico)steroids Used?

Steroids are drugs which reduce inflammation. They may clear psoriasis temporarily. Different steroids have different potencies and are available as creams, ointments, and lotions. It is strongly suggested that weaker preparations may be used on more sensitive areas of the body such as the genitals, armpits, and face while stronger preparations may be used for lesions on the scalp, elbows, knees, palms, soles, and parts of the body. Dressing may be applied to enhance the effectiveness of steroids. Corticosteroids must be used cautiously, strong steroid preparations can cause thinning of the skin, dilated blood vessels, bruising, stretch marks, and skin color changes. Stopping these medications suddenly may result in a flare-up. When used for many months, psoriasis can become resistant to the corticosteroid. Difficult-to-treat spots may be treated with an injection of a corticosteroid.

When is Anthralin Used in Psoriasis?

In tough-to-treat thick patches of psoriasis, anthralin decreases inflammation, but may itself cause irritation and pigmentation. Newer preparations and treatment methods minimize the traditional side effects of skin irritation and staining.

What are the Newer Drugs available for Localized Psoriasis?

Two new drugs available are:
- *Calcipotriene*: Effective and easy to use but expensive medication, it is useful for individuals with localized psoriasis. It is frequently combined with steroids. Best avoided on the face.
- *Retinoids*: It may be used alone or in combination with topical steroids for treatment of localized psoriasis. Women who are or may become pregnant should not use topical retinoids.

How is Light Therapy Used in Psoriasis?

Patients with psoriasis may receive light therapy treatment from artificial source at a dermatologist's clinic or in a hospital or from nature in the form of sunlight. Light therapy is a safe and effective treatment option. There are two types of light therapy:

- Ultraviolet B (UVB) therapy
- PUVA therapy

What is Ultraviolet B (UVB) Light Therapy for Psoriasis?

In UVB treatment, the skin is exposed to a wavelength of UV light called UVB, usually delivered from a chamber fitted with panel fluorescent tubes. Usually, a small spectrum of UVB is given. So, it is aptly termed narrow band UVB. This therapy may be used alone or in combination with other topical or systemic treatments. About 24 treatments over an 8-week period is usually needed for clearing. Although UVB is very safe and effective, it may be associated with side effects such as burns, freckling, and premature aging. The risk of skin cancer appears to be no greater than the risk caused by sun exposure.

What is Psoralen Plus Ultraviolet-A Therapy for Psoriasis?

PUVA stands for "psoralen + UVA"—the two components of this treatment. Psoralens are used orally (locally, if disease is localized) followed by exposure of lesions to measured amount of a type of ultraviolet light—UVA. The UVA can be delivered on the skin by special chambers or in tropics the sun may be used as the source of UVA. PUVA is used to treat extensive psoriasis and psoriasis that has not responded to other therapies. Since psoralens remain in the lens of the eye if given orally, patients must wear UVA-blocking eyeglasses when exposed to sunlight from the time the psoralen is taken until sunset that day. Clearing usually begins after approximately 25 PUVA treatments, which are given over a 2–3 month period. Keeping psoriasis under control requires about 30–40 treatments a year. PUVA treatments over a long period may increase the risk of premature aging, freckling, and skin cancer (the last being controversial).

When is Oral Treatment Required?

Oral treatment is required when psoriasis is more extensive than can comfortably be managed with topical therapy. Oral treatment is also used if topical therapy is ineffective despite a reasonable period of usage.

What are the Options Available in Systemic Therapy in Psoriasis?

Systemic therapy of psoriasis involves use of drugs which have adverse effects and so these should be always used under supervision of a trained dermatologist.

Several options are available as systemic therapy:
- Methotrexate
- Retinoids
- Cyclosporine
- Hydroxyurea
- Apremilast
- Biologics

Index

Page numbers followed by *b* refer to box, *f* refer to figure, *fc* refer to flowchart, and *t* refer to table.